SACROILIAC JOINT TECHNIQUES

Other books in this series

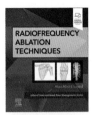

Alaa Abd-Elsayed, Radiofrequency Ablation Techniques, 1e
ISBN: 9780323870634

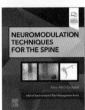

Alaa Abd-Elsayed, Neuromodulation Techniques for the Spine, 1e
ISBN: 9780323875844

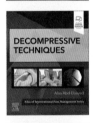

Alaa Abd-Elsayed, Decompressive Techniques, 1e
ISBN : 9780323877510

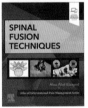

Alaa Abd-Elsayed, Spinal Fusion Techniques, 1e
ISBN: 9780323882231

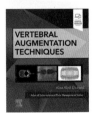

Alaa Abd-Elsayed, Vertebral Augmentation Techniques, 1e
ISBN: 9780323882262

SACROILIAC JOINT TECHNIQUES

Atlas of Interventional Pain Management Series

Alaa Abd-Elsayed, MD, MPH, CPE, FASA

Medical Director, UW Health Pain Services
Medical Director, UW Pain Clinic
Division Chief, Chronic Pain Management
Department of Anesthesiology
University of Wisconsin
Madison, Wisconsin
United States

ELSEVIER

Elsevier
1600 John F. Kennedy Blvd.
Ste 1800
Philadelphia, PA 19103-2899

SACROILIAC JOINT TECHNIQUES
Atlas of Interventional Pain Management Series
Copyright © 2024 by Elsevier Inc. All rights reserved.

ISBN: 978-0-323-87754-1

Executive Content Strategist: Michael Houston†
Senior Content Development Specialist: Malvika Shah
Publishing Services Manager: Shereen Jameel
Project Manager: Nandhini Thanga Alagu
Design Direction: Patrick C. Ferguson

Printed in India

Last digit is the print number: 9 8 7 6 5 4 3 2 1

Dedication

To my parents, wife, and my two beautiful kids Maro and George

List of Contributors

Hamid R Abbasi, MD, PhD
Chief Medical Officer, Inspired Spine
Burnsville, Minnesota
United States

Alaa Abd-Elsayed, MD, MPH, CPE, FASA
Medical Director, UW Health Pain Services
Medical Director, UW Pain Clinic
Division Chief, Chronic Pain Management
Department of Anesthesiology
University of Wisconsin
Madison, Wisconsin
United States

Ali Arastu, MD
University of Chicago Hospital
Anesthesia and Critical Care
University of Chicago, Hyde Park
Chicago, Illinois
United States

Ryan Budwany, MD, MBA, MPH
Pain Medicine
Center for Spine and Nerve
Charleston, West Virginia
United States

Ahish Chitneni, DO
Department of Rehabilitation and Regenerative
   Medicine
New York-Presbyterian Hospital—Columbia and
   Cornell
New York, New York
United States

Emmanuel Faluade, MD
Department of Anesthesiology, Perioperative Care,
   & Pain Medicine
New York University Langone Health
New York, New York
United States

George Girgis, DO
Assistant Professor of Anesthesiology
Lerner College of Medicine of Case
Western Reserve University
Staff
Pain Management Department
Anesthesiology Institute
Cleveland Clinic
Cleveland, Ohio
United states

Christopher Haddad
John Carroll University
Cleveland, Ohio
United States

Nasir Hussain, MD, MSc
Anesthesiology
The Ohio State University, Wexner Medical Center
Columbus, Ohio
United States

Meera Kirpekar, MD
Assistant Professor
Department of Anesthesiology, Perioperative Care,
   and Pain Medicine
NYU Langone
New York, New York
United States

Tariq Malik, MD
Associate Professor
Anesthesia and Critical Care
University of Chicago
Chicago, Illinois
United States

Yeshvant A. Navalgund, MD
Assistant Professor
Anesthesiology and pain medicine
West Virginia University
Morgantown, West Virginia
United States

Evan Parker, MD
Pain Management Department
Anesthesiology Institute
Cleveland Clinic Foundation
Cleveland, Ohio
United states

Divya Patel, MD
Department of Anesthesiology, Perioperative Care,
   & Pain Medicine
New York University Langone Health
New York, New York
United States

Nicholas R. Storlie
Creighton University School of Medicine
Omaha, Nebraska
United States

Timothy J. Woodin, MD
The Ohio State University
Wexner Medical Center
Department of Anesthesiology
Columbus, Ohio
United States

Christine Zaky
Loyola University, Chicago Stritch School of Medicine
Chicago, Illinois
United States

John Zaky
John Carroll University
Cleveland, Ohio
United States

Sherif Zaky, MD, MSc, PhD
Professor of Anesthesiology
Ohio University
Medical Director of Pain Management Services
Firelands Health System
Ohio, United States

Preface

The sacroiliac joint is a major contributor to symptoms of low back pain across a wide range of age groups. Sacroiliac joint pain was described decades ago, but early treatment options were limited to medical therapeutics, steroid injections, and radiofrequency ablation procedures.

Recently, the sacroiliac joint has been identified as an anatomical location amenable to interventional procedures that result in treatment of sacroiliac joint pain syndromes.

Novel interventions include neuromodulation and joint fusion. Diverse pain management systems for both neuromodulation and joint fusion serve to broaden the available treatment options available to the interventional pain physician. With these advancements, there remains a need to master surgical techniques and skills to facilitate the safe and efficient performance of these procedures.

This atlas provides a comprehensive guide to the traditional and advanced procedures utilized in the treatment of sacroiliac joint pain conditions. The book leverages liberal utilization of high-quality anatomical and radiographic figures to provide a comprehensive guide to performing procedures aimed at alleviating sacroiliac joint pain syndromes.

I would like to thank the authors and publisher for their efforts and dedication to writing and producing this atlas that I hope will be guide for physicians all over the world.

Alaa Abd-Elsayed, MD, MPH, CPE, FASA

Contents

Chapter 1

Anatomy of the Sacroiliac Joint

John Zaky, Christopher Haddad, and Sherif Zaky

The sacroiliac joint (SIJ) is a highly complex joint that provides stability and support to the upper body (Fig. 1.1). The specific structure and tightness of the fibrous apparatus of the SIJ results in its limited mobility. The importance of the SIJ as a stress reliever between the trunk and lower limbs has been emphasized.[1] This joint ensures that the pelvic girdle is not a sold ring of bones that can easily break under routine stresses it might be subject to. The SIJ is known to be the largest axial spinal joint in the body and is approximately 17.5 cm^2.[2] The SIJ is a true diarthrodial joint that is more mobile in youth than later in life. The female pelvis is also more mobile to accommodate pregnancy and parturition.[3,4] This joint has at multiple junctures a fibrous joint capsule that contains a thick synovial fluid, cartilaginous surfaces, and numerous ligamentous connections. It is different from other synovial joints in that the iliac articulation is made of fibrocartilage rather than hyaline cartilage.

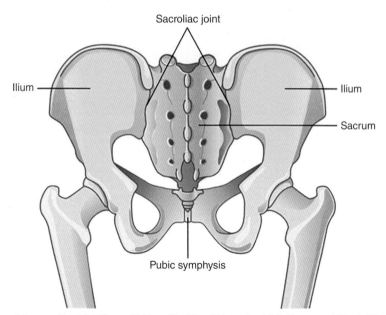

Fig. 1.1 Bony anatomy of the sacroiliac joint. (Source: Waldman SD. *Atlas of Interventional Pain Management*. 5th ed. Philadelphia: Elsevier; 2021.)

Bony Anatomy

There is great variance in shape and size of the bony anatomy of the SIJ among individuals[5] (Fig. 1.2). From infancy to adulthood, notable changes in the joint occur.[6] The articular surface of the sacrum is generally concave, and the iliac surface is predominantly convex. The SIJ has numerous ridges and grooves compared with a typical synovial joint. This characteristic of the joint minimizes movement, further enhancing stability.[7] The ventral aspect of the SIJ frequently has defects that allows fluid in the joint to leak out to the surrounding structures.[8]

Sacralization, or fusion of the fifth lumbar vertebrae into the body of the sacrum, occurs in about 6% of American adults.[9] Fusion between the L5 and S1 vertebrae can occur at one or more locations, such as between transverse processes, vertebral bodies, or facet joints. Accessory SIJs have been described as extracapsular articulations for biomechanical enhancement.[10]

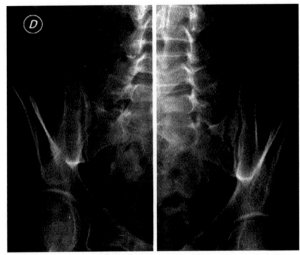

Fig. 1.2 Fluoroscopic anatomy of the sacroiliac joint. (Source: Waldman SD. *Atlas of Interventional Pain Management*. 5th ed. Philadelphia: Elsevier; 2021.)

Ligaments and Muscles Supporting the Sacroiliac Joint

The SIJ is mainly designed to support stability and weight bearing with only small degrees of rotation and translation allowed.[7,11] Joint stability is enforced by multiple ligaments that include the anterior sacroiliac ligament (ASL), posterior sacroiliac ligament (PSL), sacrospinous ligament (SSL), sacrotuberous ligament (STL), and interosseous ligament (which is considered the strongest)[2,4] (Figs. 1.3 and 1.4). The interosseous sacroiliac ligament encloses the axial joint and fills the spaces dorsal and caudal to the synovial joint. It has the most extensive bony attachment and volume

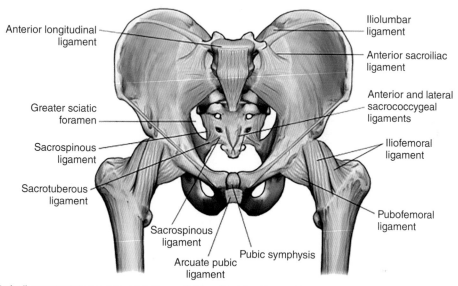

Fig. 1.3 **The anterior ligaments of the sacroiliac joint.** (Source: Waldman SD. *Atlas of Interventional Pain Management.* 5th ed. Philadelphia: Elsevier; 2021.)

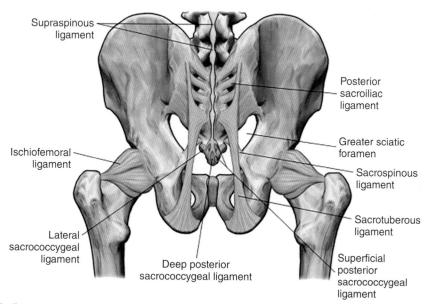

Fig. 1.4 **The posterior ligaments of the sacroiliac joint.** (Source: Waldman SD. *Atlas of Interventional Pain Management.* 5th ed. Philadelphia: Elsevier; 2021.)

among all sacroiliac ligaments.[12] The axial joint is therefore difficult to access because of the irregular contour, extensive fibrous apparatus, and individual variations. Whereas the PSL has the most influence on the joint mobility, the ASL has very limited effect.[13] The iliolumbar (IL) ligament is a large fan-shaped structure that extends from the transverse processes of the lower two lumbar vertebrae to the iliac crest and the SIJ capsule.[14] The main function of the IL ligament is to restrict movements at the lumbosacral junction, especially side bending.[15]

The joint is also supported by a group of muscles, including the gluteus maximus, gluteus medius, piriformis, biceps femoris, and latissimus dorsi via thoracolumbar fascia and erector spinae. The psoas major muscle is immediately anterior to the SIJ.

Innervation of the Sacroiliac Joint

The innervation of the sacroiliac joint is controversial and remains a topic of debate. Recent literature suggests that lateral branches of the S1 to S3 dorsal rami compose the major innervation to the posterior SI joint with some suggestion that dorsal rami components as extensive as L3 to S4 may contribute to joint innervation[2] (Fig. 1.5). The innervation of the anterior joint is likewise uncertain, with recent literature indicating contributions from different combinations of

the ventral rami of L2 to S2[16] and older literature suggesting possible contributions from the obturator and superior gluteal nerves.[17] A successful attenuation of SIJ pain using neurotomy of the L5 dorsal ramus and lateral branches of S1 to S3 was reported by Patel et al.[18] in 2012. Dissection and fluoroscopic imaging of small wires placed on the lateral branches of the dorsal sacral plexus demonstrated small fibers entering the medical and inferior boundaries of the SIJ.[19] The axons of these nerves were found to include C-fibers and possibly A-delta fibers.[20]

REFERENCES

1. Lovejoy CO. Evolution of human walking. *Sci Am.* 1988;259(5): 118-125.
2. Cohen SP. Sacroiliac joint pain: a comprehensive review of anatomy, diagnosis, and treatment [review]. *Anesth Analg.* 2005; 101(5):1440-1453.
3. Bernard Jr TN. The sacroiliac joint syndrome: pathophysiology, diagnosis, and management. In: Frymoyer JW, ed. *The Adult Spine. Principles and Practice.* New York: Raven; 1991: 2107-2130.
4. Goode A, Hegedus EJ, Sizer P, Brismee JM, Linberg A, Cook CE. Three-dimensional movements of the sacroiliac joint: a systematic review of the literature and assessment of clinical utility. *J Man Manip Ther.* 2008;16(1):25-38.
5. Schunke GB. The anatomy and development of the Sacro-Iliac joint in man. *Anat Rec.* 1938;72:313-331.
6. Bowen V, Cassidy JD. Macroscopic and microscopic anatomy of the sacroiliac joint from embryonic life to the eighth decade. *Spine (Phila Pa 1976).* 1981;6:620-628.

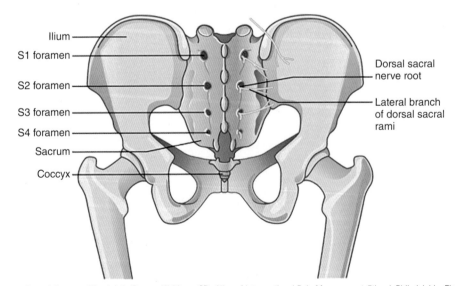

Fig. 1.5 Innervation of the sacroiliac joint. (Source: Waldman SD. *Atlas of Interventional Pain Management.* 5th ed. Philadelphia: Elsevier; 2021.)

7. Forst SL, Wheeler MT, Fortin JD, et al. The sacroiliac joint. Anatomy, physiology and clinical significance. *Pain Physician.* 2006; 9:1533-1539.
8. Fortin JD, Kissling RO, O'Connor BL, et al. Sacroiliac joint innervation and pain. *Am J Orthop.* 1999;28(12):687-690.
9. Tague RG. High assimilation of the sacrum in a sample of American skeletons: prevalence, pelvic size, and obstetrical and evolutionary implications. *Am J Phys Anthropol.* 2009;138:429-438.
10. Trotter M. Accessory sacroiliac articulations in East African skeletons. *Am J Phys Anthropol.* 1964;22:137-141.
11. Egund N, Olsson TH, Schmid H, et al. Movements in the sacroiliac joints demonstrated with roentgen stereophotogrammetric analysis. *Acta Radiol Diagn.* 1978;19:833-845.
12. Steinke H, Hammer N, Slowik V, et al. Novel insights into the sacroiliac joint ligaments. *Spine (Phila Pa 1976).* 2010;35:257-263.
13. Vrahas M, Hern TC, Diangelo D, et al. Ligamentous contributions to pelvic stability. *Orthopedics.* 1995;18:271-274.
14. Pool-Goudzwaard AL, Kleinrensink GJ, Snijders CJ, et al. The sacroiliac part of the iliolumbar ligament. *J Anat.* 2001;199: 457-463.
15. Leong JC, Luk KD, Chow DH, et al. The biomechanical functions of the iliolumbar ligament in maintaining stability of the lumbosacral junction. *Spine (Phila Pa 1976).* 1987;12: 669-674.
16. Forst SL, Wheeler MT, Fortin JD, Vilensky JA. The sacroiliac joint: anatomy, physiology and clinical significance [review]. *Pain Physician.* 2006;9(1):61-67.
17. Pitkin HC, Pheasant HC. Sacrarthrogenic telalgia I: a study of referred pain. *J Bone Joint Surg.* 1936;18:111-133.
18. Patel N, Gross A, Brown L, et al. A randomized, placebo-controlled study to assess the efficacy of lateral branch neurotomy for chronic sacroiliac joint pain. *Pain Med.* 2012;13: 383-398.
19. Yin W, Willard F, Carreiro J, et al. Sensory stimulation guided sacroiliac joint radiofrequency neurotomy: technique based on neuroanatomy of the dorsal sacral plexus. *Spine (Phila Pa 1976).* 2003;28:2419-2425.
20. Ikeda R. Innervation of the sacroiliac joint. Macroscopical and histological studies. *Nippon Ika Daigaku Zasshi.* 1991;58:587-596.

Chapter 2

Surgical Instruments

Ali Arastu and Tariq Malik

Introduction

Surgical instruments are the tools of the trade. Just like any in any other trade or manual job, there are a number of surgical instruments that have been designed to perform specific tasks. Surgical instruments have been found dating back to prehistoric times when they were made up of stone or animal bones. The 19th century saw the development of anesthesia and antiseptic techniques, which was the start of modern surgery. The 20th century saw the growth of endoscopic techniques along with ever increasing role of laser and ultrasound devices in the operating room (OR). The majority of the surgical tools are still made from stainless steel, which makes them resistant to corrosion.

Each surgical instrument is designed and built for a specific use. Using it for any other purpose will damage or shorten the life of the instrument. There are some basic rules and etiquettes of handling the instruments in the OR. The surgical technician is there to help you. The technician ensures the instruments are safely held and placed before, during, and after surgery. Instruments should not be tossed or dropped. Heavy items and instruments should not be placed on top of the patient or on other instruments. Careless or mishandlings is not only damaging to the instruments but can hurt others.

Parts of an Instrument[1]

The design of the instrument depends on its purpose. Overall, each instrument is constructed around a basic design, which is modified to serve its function. The components of basic design are *handles*, *ratchet*, *shanks*, *joints*, *jaws* or *blades*, and *tips*.

The *handle* is where the user holds the instrument; it is connected to the *jaw* or *blade* via the *shank*. The jaw or the blade is the functional part of the instrument. The *joint* connects the two halves of the instrument and acts as a fulcrum. The *ratchets* attached to the shanks give the instrument a locking function. The *blade* and *tip* shape give the instrument its functionality. The *shanks* determine size of the instrument while maintaining function (Fig. 2.1).

This chapter reviews basic surgical instruments commonly used in interventional pain procedures. Figures of each instrument are followed by a brief description of the instrument and its uses. The details of how to handle or use the instrument is not included, which is best learned with hands-on experience with a proctor.

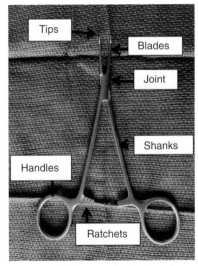

Fig. 2.1 Basic parts of an instrument.

List of Instruments

ELECTROSURGICAL PEN[1,2]

Other Names

Bovie, bi- or monopolar, cautery

Category

Energy systems

Description

This is a disposable instrument that comes packaged with a blade tip and a holster. It has a high-powered and high-frequency generator that produces a radio-frequency spark between a probe and the surgical site that causes localized heating and damage to the tissue. The current can be activated by a button on the pencil or with a foot pedal (Fig. 2.2).

Use(s)

A surgical device used to incise tissue, destroy tissue through desiccation, and control bleeding by causing coagulation of blood.

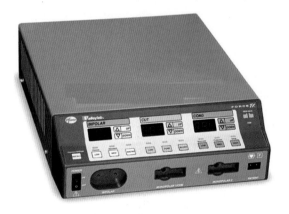

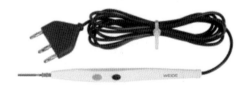

Fig. 2.2 Electrocautery generator and pen.

Instrument Insight

The device was invented by Dr. WT Bovie. He made the device in 1926 when he heard Dr. Cushing inability to operate on tumors that were bloody during dissection. Cushing published his use of electrosurgical technique in a series of 500 cases. The electrosurgical principle is often incorrectly referred as electrocautery. In electrosurgery, the generator sends an alternating current into the body; the current then heats up the tissue. The tip of the instrument never gets heated. Although the electrocautery process involves heating up the device and then transmitting the heat to the tissue, the current never enters the body. The wave form of the current allows the surgeon to either cut or coagulate the tissue. In cut mode, the generator produces continuous low-voltage standard waveform. This high, intense, continuous energy vaporizes the tissue, resulting in a clean cut. In coagulate mode, the generator delivers high-voltage, low-current waves intermittently. This causes desiccation and seals the bleeding vessels. The instrument allows the surgeon to operate efficiently and precisely and with minimal blood loss. Cut mode is less damaging to the tissue than coagulation mode. Excessive use can cause tissue charring and damage blood supply to the tissue, which can both contribute to poor healing, infection, and seroma formation.

The user can operate in monopolar mode or bipolar mode. In monopolar mode, an active electrode concentrates the current to the surgical site, and a dispersive electrode channel (a grounding pad) takes the current away from the patient. The grounding pad should be placed close to the operative site on the ipsilateral side of the surgical field and away from any metallic implant. The pad should completely contact the skin. Uneven contact because of hair, bony prominence, or scar can cause skin damage. In bipolar mode, both the active and return electrodes are located at the surgical site, and there is no need for the grounding pad (returning electrode). The principle of electrosurgery relies on the principle of high-frequency electrical current entering the tissue; therefore, the best results are obtained when electrode tips are kept clean. A scratch pad is provided to remove charred blood or tissue from the electrode tip.

Caution

The tip of the pencil becomes hot after extended use. When not in use, place the pencil in a holster to prevent burning the drapes or the patient.

STRAIGHT HALSTEAD[1,2]

Other Name

Mosquito forceps

Category

Clamping and occluding

Description

It is a small curved or straight clamp with fine tips and horizontal serrations that run the length of the jaws. It is used to occlude bleeding vessels before coagulating them with Bovie or ligating them. Halsted forceps are similar to Hartman forceps in shape and function except that Halsted forceps are lighter and a little bigger in size, ranging from 5.5 to 8.25 inches in length (Fig. 2.3).

Use(s)

Used as a hemostatic agent to compress smaller vessels that regulates blood flow. Also used with suture boots to tag delicate Prolene sutures in vascular procedures.

Instrument Insight

The forceps have a 5-inch working length. They are much smaller than a Crile or Kelly forceps.

CRILE FORCEPS[1,2]

Other Names

Hemostat, snap, clamp, stat

Category

Clamping and occluding

Description

The forceps have horizontal serrations on the entire length of the jaw. The jaws are half the length of the shank. Crile forceps have finger rings and locking ratchets to secure the tissue and vessels (Fig. 2.4).

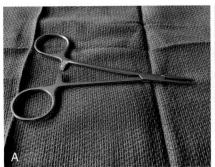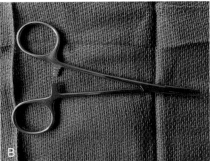

Fig. 2.3 **A** and **B,** Straight Halstead forceps.

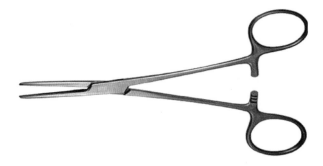

Fig. 2.4 Crile forceps.

Use(s)

Atraumatic and nontoothed clamp used to grasp tissue or vessels that will be tied off. It is also used in blunt dissection.

Instrument Insight

The curved Crile is the most commonly used clamp forceps. Kelly forceps are a larger size variation of hemostat with similar function.

KELLY FORCEPS[1,2]
Other Names

Hemostat, Kelly clamp

Category

Clamping and occluding

Description

Very similar to Crile forceps, but Kelly forceps have a longer jaw for clamping. The jaw is only half serrated. Kelly forceps have finger rings and locking ratchets to secure the tissue and vessels (Fig. 2.5).

Use(s)

Used for occluding bleeders before cauterization or ligation. Also, it is used in blunt dissections.

ROCHESTER-PEAN FORCEPS[1,2]
Other Names

Pean, Mayo, Kelly-Pean forceps, Big Kelly

Category

Camping and occluding

Description

The Rochester-Pean forceps have both straight and curved styles with fully serrated jaws. They have a built-in ratchet mechanism that is able to hold objects firm. It is heavier built and comes in different sizes from 5.5 to 8 inches (Fig. 2.6).

Use(s)

A hemostat used to control bleeding. It is used to occlude larger blood vessels and tissue before ligation. Seen used more in deeper wounds or heavier tissue.

Instrumental Insight

Sometimes referred to as the "big hemostat" or "big Kelly"

CARMALT FORCEPS[1,2]
Other Names

Carmalt; Rochester-Carmalt Forceps; big, curved forceps; "stars and stripes hemostat"

Category

Clamping and occluding

Description

Carmalt forceps have longitudinal serrations the entire length of the jaw, and the tips are cross-serrated. It comes with either straight or curved jaws. Forceps have ring handles and a ratchet for a secure grip. These are large, crushing hemostatic forceps used for clamping blood vessels and large tissues or ligating pedicles. The textured blades,

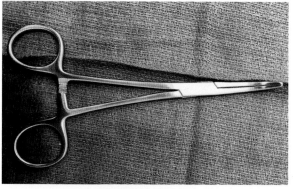

Fig. 2.5 Kelly forceps.

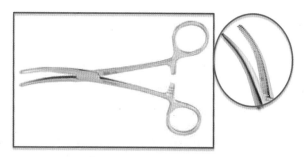

Fig. 2.6 Rochester-Pean forceps.

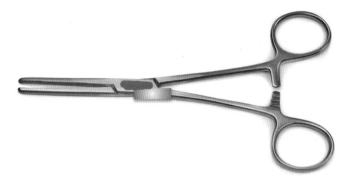

Fig. 2.7 Carmalt forceps.

along with the scissor-like ratchet handles, ensure a strong grip. The size varies from 16 to 20 cm (Fig. 2.7).

Use(s)

A heavy tip and longitudinal serrations provide grip on heavy tissue and stop blood flow of large vessels.

MIXTER FORCEPS[1,2]

Other Names

Right-angle forceps, Gemini forceps, Lahey forceps, obtuse clamp, ureter clamp

Category

Clamping and occluding

Description

Mixter forceps are available in multiple lengths and have serrations the entire length of the jaw. Forceps have straight shanks, fully serrated jaws, and right-angle tips.

Use(s)

Used for working in obscured surgical sites. They are most frequently used for clamping, dissection, or grasping tissue. Also commonly used to place a tie or vessel loop under and around a vessel or duct. It enables the surgeon to grasp the ligature or loop and pull it up and around the structure to either ligate or retract (Fig. 2.8).

PLAIN ADSON TISSUE FORCEPS[1,2]

Other Name

Adson dressing forceps

Category

Grasping and holding

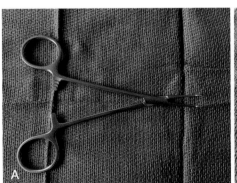
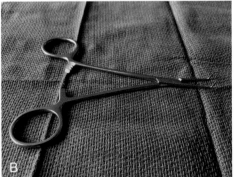

Fig. 2.8 A and **B**, Mixter forceps.

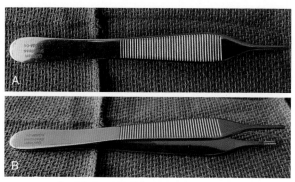

Fig. 2.9 **A** and **B,** Plain Adson tissue forceps.

Description

Narrow tips with horizontal serrations (Fig. 2.9)

Use(s)

Used for holding and manipulating delicate tissue.

Instrument Insight

Tips can have different configurations. All the Adson tissue forceps are the same size and shape. The only difference is the inner tips.

TOOTHED ADSON TISSUE FORCEPS[1,2]

Other Names

Adsons with teeth, rat tooth

Category

Grasping and holding

Description

Narrow tips with two small teeth on one side and one small tooth on the other side (Fig. 2.10)

Use(s)

Used to align edges of the wound during stapling or when Steri-Strips are placed.

Instrument Insight

Tips can have different configurations. All the Adson tissue forceps are the same size and shape. The only difference is the inner tips.

BROWN ADSON TISSUE FORCEPS[1,2]

Other Name

Brown forceps

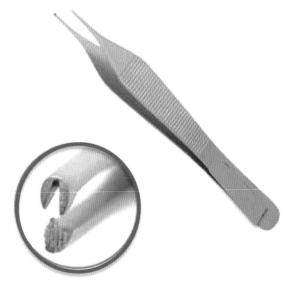

Fig. 2.10 Toothed Adson tissue forceps.

Category

Grasping and holding

Description

Narrow tips with two rows of multiple teeth on each side. The teeth interlock when closed (Fig. 2.11).

Use(s)

Used for grasping superficial delicate tissue.

Instrument Insight

Tips can have different configurations. All the Adson tissue forceps are the same size and shape. The only difference is the inner tips.

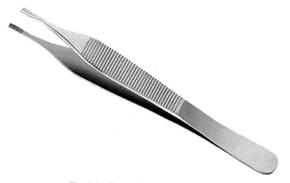

Fig. 2.11 Brown Adson tissue forceps.

STRAIGHT MAYO SCISSORS[1,2]

Other Name

Suture scissors

Category

Cutting and dissecting

Description

Heavy scissors with straight blades, made from stainless steel or titanium material. It comes in standard size (6 inches) or as extra. The tips are rounder than Metzenbaum and look blunter (Fig. 2.12).

Use(s)

Designed for cutting body tissues near the surface of a wound and are also used for cutting sutures.

Instrument Insight

When cutting sutures, use the tips of the scissors.

Caution

The blades of scissors should be inspected for dents or nicks that will not allow for smooth cutting. It is important to also check the screw to ensure it is fully tightened to prevent it from dropping into the wound.

CURVED MAYO SCISSORS[1,2]

Other Name

Heavy tissue scissors

Category

Cutting and dissecting

Description

Heavy scissors with curved blades

Use(s)

Used to cut thick tissues and to dissect or undermine heavy fibrous tissue

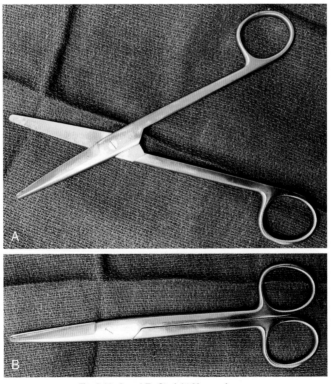

Fig. 2.12 A and **B,** Straight Mayo scissors.

Instrument Insight

Mayo scissors used for dissection are placed in tissue with the tips closed. The scissors are then opened so that the tips open and spread out the tissue during the dissection process (Fig. 2.13).

METZENBAUM SCISSORS[1,2]
Other Names

Metz scissors, tissue scissors

Category

Cutting and dissecting

Description

Lighter scissors. Have a longer handle to blade distance. Can have blunt or sharp tips (Fig. 2.14).

Use(s)

Used for cutting delicate tissue and for blunt dissection.

Instrument Insight

It should only be used to cut heavy or thick tissue. It is meant for delicate tissue dissection or finding tissue plans. If used to cut sutures, the blades can become dull and not function properly.

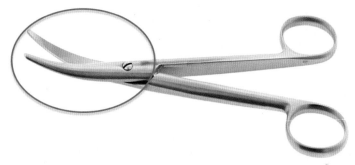

Fig. 2.13 Curved Mayo scissors.

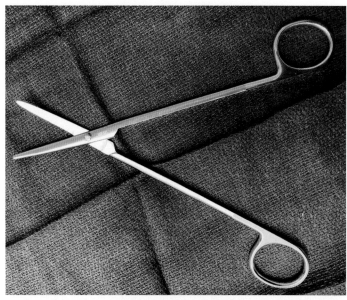

Fig. 2.14 Metzenbaum scissors.

LISTER BANDAGE SCISSORS[1,2]

Other Name

Bandage scissors

Category

Cutting and dissecting

Description

Jaws of scissors are angled with the lower blade being slightly longer. Ring handles can be equal in size or with one ring larger (Fig. 2.15).

Use(s)

Scissors are used for sizing dressings and removing circumferential bandages. The tip of the lower blade features a flattened blunt nodule that is intended to slide between bandages and skin without harming the skin.

Instrument Insight

Can be used in cesarean section to open the uterus without causing inadvertent injury to the baby

WIRE SCISSORS[1,2]

Other Name

Wire cutters

Category

Cutting and dissecting

Description

Curved scissors. Blades with fine serrations. Has a circular notch in the inner jaws for cutting wires (Fig. 2.16).

Use(s)

Cut small gauge wires and sutures.

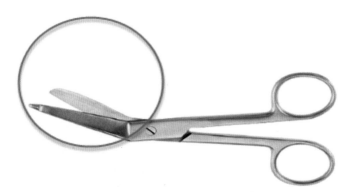

Fig. 2.15 Lister bandage scissors.

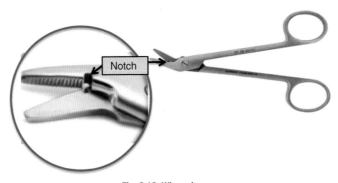

Notch

Fig. 2.16 Wire scissors.

Instrument Insight

The serrations are intended to facilitate grasping the item being cut. When the wire is placed inside the notch, it gives the scissors the ability to exert additional pressure to cut heavier gauge wire.

NO. 3 KNIFE HANDLE[1,2]

Other Names

No. 3 scalpel handle, no. 3 handle

Category

Cutting and dissecting

Description

A no. 3 handle holds blades 10, 11, 12, and 15. It has grooves to assist in a better grip and to avoid slippage. Its long handle is used to help make deep cuts within a wound (Fig. 2.17).

Use(s)

Knife handles hold various blades to make a scalpel. When a handle is attached to blades, it is used to make straight, long cuts.

Instrument Insight

Because skin is not sterile, after skin incision is made, the scalpel should be removed from Mayo stand, because it is unsterile. It is only to be reused to incise the skin.

Caution

Never retrieve a scalpel from the surgeon's hands. Wait until the surgeon places it in the neutral zone before picking it up. Never use your fingers to unload or load a knife blade from the handle. A needle holder should be used when manipulating the blade.

NO. 7 KNIFE HANDLE[1,2]

Other Names

No. 7 scalpel handle, no. 7 handle

Category

Cutting and dissecting

Description

A no. 7 knife handle holds blades 10, 11, 12, and 15. It is more rounded in shape and contains a thin neck toward the top, similar to a writing pen (Fig. 2.18).

Use(s)

Used when precision cutting is needed in a confined space or deep wound.

Caution

Never retrieve a scalpel from the surgeon's hands. Wait until the surgeon places it in the neutral zone before picking it up. Never use your fingers to unload or load a knife blade from the handle. A needle holder should be used when manipulating the blade.

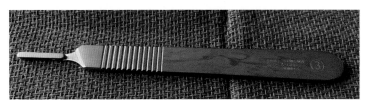

Fig. 2.17 No. 3 knife handle.

Fig. 2.18 No. 7 knife handle.

NO. 10 BLADE[1,2]

Category

Cutting and dissecting

Description

Curved blade and said to have a "belly." Sharpest area on the blade is at the apex of the curve of the belly (Fig. 2.19).

Use(s)

Used for making large incisions through skin and subcutaneous tissues, as in the case of a laparotomy.

Instrument Insight

Always use a needle holder when manipulating the blade. To load the scalpel, line up the grooves on the handle with the opening on the blade. When the angle of the blade matches the angle of the handle, advance the blade onto the handle until it clicks in place. A scalpel blade is a single-patient use item.

Caution

Never use fingers to manipulate the blade. Always use a needle holder.

NO. 11 BLADE[1,2]

Category

Cutting and dissecting

Description

Angled cutting edge that ascends to a sharp point (Fig. 2.20)

Use(s)

Used for puncturing the skin like a stab wound. Commonly used for placing a large cannula or initiating the opening of a vessel. It's often included in central line or other procedural equipment kits. It is used to make a precise or a sharply angled incision.

Instrument Insight

A scalpel blade is a single-patient use item. No. 11 blade is commonly loaded onto the no. 7 handle.

Caution

Never use fingers to manipulate the blade. Always use a needle holder.

NO. 15 BLADE[1,2]

Category

Cutting and dissecting

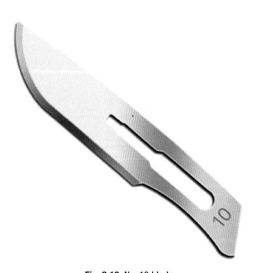

Fig. 2.19 No. 10 blade.

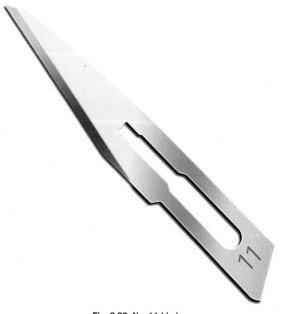

Fig. 2.20 No. 11 blade.

Description

Blade with a small, curved cutting edge (Fig. 2.21)

Use(s)

It is ideal for making short and precise incisions.

Instrument Insight

A scalpel blade is a single-patient use item. It is usually used in pediatric or plastic surgery. It can also be used for a stab incision for placing a large cannula through the skin.

Caution

Never use fingers to manipulate the blade. Always use a needle holder.

NO. 4 KNIFE HANDLE[1,2]

Other Names

No. 4 scalpel handle, no. 4 handle

Category

Cutting and dissecting

Description

A no. 4 handle holds blades that start with digit 2 such as 20, 21, 22, 23, 24, and 25. It has a larger tip to accommodate the larger blades (Fig. 2.22).

Use(s)

When attached to the blade, it is used to create a larger and/or deeper incision in heavy tissue areas.

Instrument Insight

Because the skin is not sterile, after skin incision is made, the scalpel should be removed from the Mayo stand. It is only to be reused to incise the skin.

Caution

Never retrieve a scalpel from the surgeon's hands. Wait until the surgeon places it in the neutral zone before

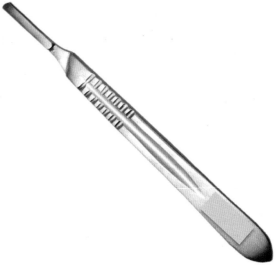

Fig. 2.22 No. 4 knife handle.

picking it up. Never use your fingers to unload or load a knife blade from the handle. A needle holder should be used when manipulating the blade.

NO. 20 BLADE[1,2]

Category

Cutting and dissecting

Description

The blade has a larger body with a curved cutting edge at the tip (Fig. 2.23).

Use(s)

It is used to create a larger and/or deeper incision in heavy tissue areas and bone.

Instrument Insight

A scalpel blade is a single-patient use item.

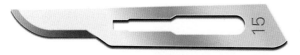

Fig. 2.21 No. 15 blade.

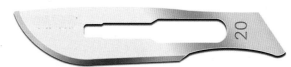

Fig. 2.23 No. 20 blade.

Caution

Never use fingers to manipulate the blade. Always use a needle holder.

TOOTHED TISSUE FORCEPS[1,2]

Other Names

Semken tissue forceps, rat tooth, tissue forceps with teeth

Category

Grasping and holding

Description

Forceps that have teeth at the end of the tip. One side of the tip has two teeth, the other side has one tooth, and they fit between one another when closed (Fig. 2.24).

Use(s)

Used for grasping moderate to heavy tissue.

DEBAKEY TISSUE FORCEPS[1,2]

Other Names

Debakey's, Debakes

Category

Grasping and holding

Description

A large forceps that have a distinct coarsely ribbed grip panel. An atraumatic forceps with an elongated, narrowed blunt tip (Fig. 2.25).

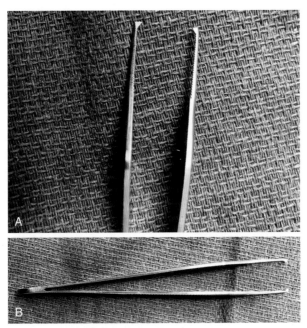

Fig. 2.24 **A** and **B,** Toothed tissue forceps.

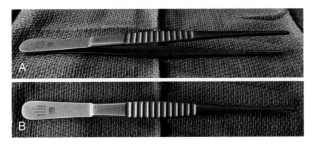

Fig. 2.25 **A** and **B,** Debakey tissue forceps.

Use(s)

It is used for atraumatic tissue grasping during dissection. It is commonly used in cardiac, vascular, and gastrointestinal procedures.

Instrument Insight

It is considered a vascular tissue forceps but is commonly used in all specialty areas because these forceps allow one to securely grip tissue without causing damage.

BONNEY TISSUE FORCEPS[1,2]
Other Names

Victor Bonney forceps, Victors

Category

Grasping and holding

Description

Forceps with a tapered serrated tip and teeth. Handle of forceps includes a comfortable grip (Fig. 2.26).

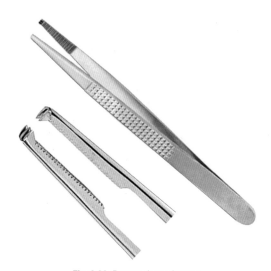

Fig. 2.26 Bonney tissue forceps.

Use(s)

Forceps are used to grasp heavy tissue or bone.

FERRIS-SMITH TISSUE FORCEPS[1,2]
Other Name

Big ugly's

Category

Grasping and holding

Description

Forceps with a wide section of the handle for greater control. The tips are slightly wider with dual teeth and serration for secure grip (Fig. 2.27).

Use(s)

Heavyweight forceps used to grasp heavy tissue.

SINGLEY TISSUE FORCEPS[1,2]
Other Name

Tuttle thoracic tissue forceps

Category

Grasping and holding

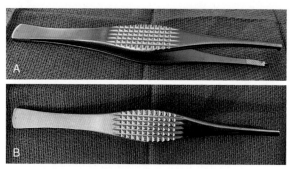

Fig. 2.27 A and B, Ferris-Smith tissue forceps.

Description

Designed with serrated loop tips. Includes a rigid handle that allows good grip for the user (Fig. 2.28).

Use(s)

Used for grasping delicate tissue such as intestinal tissue. Also used to grasp dressing materials and sponges.

RUSSIAN TISSUE FORCEPS[1,2]

Other Names

Star forceps, Russian star forceps, Russians

Category

Grasping and holding

Description

Forceps with a wide, rounded head and teeth around the rim (Fig. 2.29)

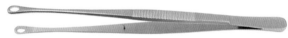

Fig. 2.28 Singley tissue forceps.

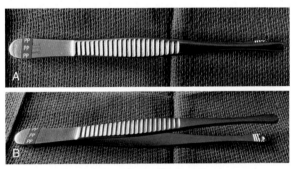

Fig. 2.29 A and **B,** Russian tissue forceps.

Use(s)

Used during wound closure or grasping dense tissues

TOWEL CLIP (PENETRATING)[1,2]

Other Names

Backhaus towel clip, Roeder towel clip, Jones towel clip.

Category

Grasping and holding

Description

A ratcheted instrument with curved, sharp jaws (Fig. 2.30)

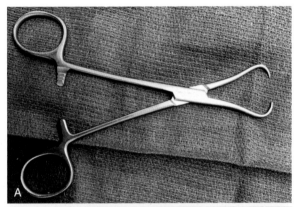

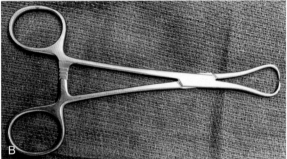

Fig. 2.30 A and **B,** Towel clip (penetrating).

Use(s)

Used to secure towels and surgical drapes during procedure.

Caution

When clipping towels together, be careful not to pierce the patient's skin.

TOWEL CLIP (NONPENETRATING)[1,2]

Other Name

Atraumatic towel clamp

Category

Grasping and holding

Description

Many different types and sizes. Can be metal or plastic. Nonpenetrating tip (Fig. 2.31).

Use(s)

Often used to attach Bovie and suction to the drapes.

Use(s)

When clipping towels together, be careful to avoid the patient's skin.

FOERSTER SPONGE FORCEPS[1,2]

Other Names

Fletcher sponge forceps, sponge stick forceps, ring forceps

Category

Grasping and holding

Description

Features oval tips with serrations. Ratchet handle helps to hold sponges firmly (Fig. 2.32).

Use(s)

Used to hold sponges during procedure. Helps with grasping tissue. Used commonly in obstetric procedures for removing uterine contents.

Instrument Insight

A sponge stick is made by folding a 4 × 4 Raytex and attaching it to the ring forceps.

ALLIS FORCEPS[1,2]

Category

Grasping and holding

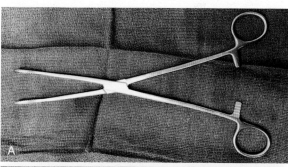
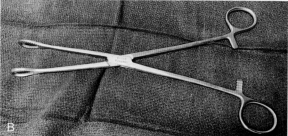

Fig. 2.32 A and **B,** Foerster sponge forceps.

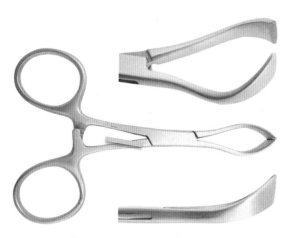

Fig. 2.31 Towel clip (nonpenetrating).

Description

Forceps with an interlocking tooth pattern on the distal tip. Has a built-in ratchet mechanism (Fig. 2.33).

Use(s)

Used to hold or grasp heavy tissue.

Instrument Insight

Allis can cause damage to tissue, so it is often used in tissue about to be removed.

BABCOCK FORCEPS[1,2]

Category

Grasping and holding

Description

Finger ring, with ratchet, nonperforating forceps (Fig. 2.34).

Use(s)

Used to hold and encircle delicate tissue such as ureters, fallopian tubes, bowel, ovaries, and appendix.

Instrument Insight

Similar to Allis forceps, although considered less traumatic because of their wider, rounded grasping surface.

KOCHER FORCEPS[1,2]

Other Names

Koch forceps, Ochsner forceps

Category

Grasping and holding

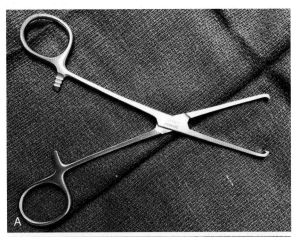

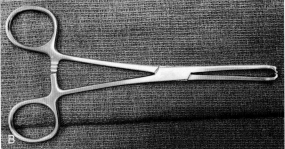

Fig. 2.33 Allis forceps.

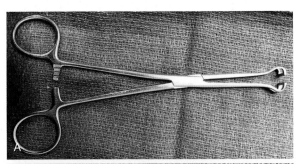

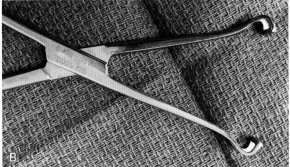

Fig. 2.34 A and B, Babcock forceps.

Description

Forceps with horizontal serrations the entire length of the jaw. Also includes teeth to ensure a firm grip on the tissue being held (Fig. 2.35).

Use(s)

A heavy instrument used to aggressively grasp medium to heavy tissue or occlude heavy and dense vessels.

ARMY-NAVY RETRACTORS[1,2]

Other Names

Army's, Navy's, US retractor

Category

Retracting and exposing

Description

Double-ended retractor with a fenestrated handle. Blades at each end are angled 90 degrees and have a

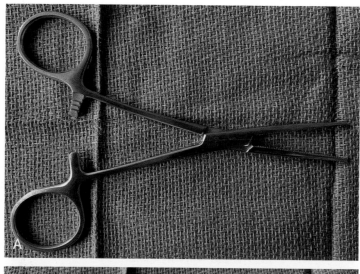

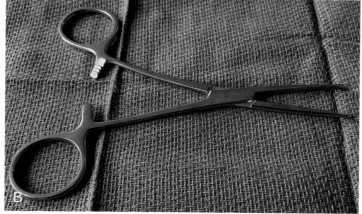

Fig. 2.35 A and **B,** Kocher forceps.

slightly curved, rounded lip. The blades face in the same direction (Fig. 2.36).

Use(s)

Used to retract superficial incisions to allow better exposure.

RICHARDSON FORCEPS[1,2]

Other Names

"Rich forceps," "Rich retractor"

Category

Retracting and exposing

Description

A Richardson retractor is 9.5-inch-long retractor that comes in various forms. The blade size varies in depth and width to suit different surgical needs, but the length tends be the same. The curved blade is used to retract soft tissue. The handle part of the instrument comes in three shapes: a grip handle, a lamb handle, or a standard hollow loop handle (Fig. 2.37).

Use(s)

It is most often used to retract abdominal or chest incisions. Used for holding back multiple layers of deep tissue. This is one of the most common retractors used in general surgery.

GOELET RETRACTOR[1,2]

Other Name

Bolt retractor

Category

Retracting and exposing

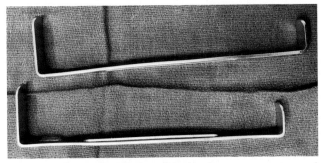

Fig. 2.36 Army-Navy retractors.

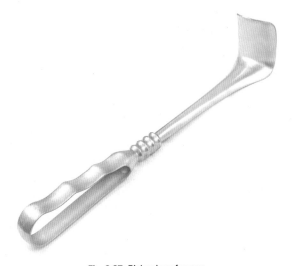

Fig. 2.37 Richardson forceps.

Description

Double-ended instrument that has smooth, cup-shaped curved blades on each end with a crescent-shaped lip. One end is longer than the other (Fig. 2.38).

Use(s)

Used to retract superficial incisions to allow better exposure.

SENN RETRACTOR[1,2]

Other Name

Cat paw retractor

Category

Retracting and exposing

Description

Double-ended retractors: one end is L shaped, and the other end has three bent prongs (Fig. 2.39).

Use(s)

Used for retraction of skin edges and deeper tissues of small incisions.

MURPHY RETRACTOR[1,2]

Other Name

Rake retractor

Category

Retracting and exposing

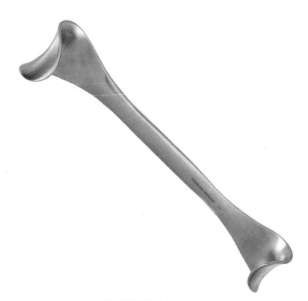

Fig. 2.38 Goelet retractor.

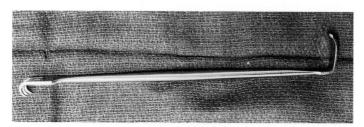

Fig. 2.39 Senn retractor.

Description

Unique fenestrated loop handle and finger grips that provides grip and maneuverability (Fig. 2.40). Prongs can either be sharp or blunt.

Use(s)

Used to retract superficial skin edges for better visibility

VOLKMAN RETRACTOR[1,2]

Other Names

Rake retractor, Israel retractor

Category

Retracting and exposing

Description

Prongs are curved and can either be blunt or sharp. Handle has a teardrop opening (Fig. 2.41).

Use(s)

Used to retract superficial skin edges for better visibility.

RIBBON RETRACTOR[1,2]

Other Name

Malleable retractor

Category

Retracting and exposing

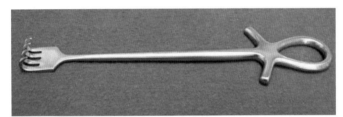

Fig. 2.40 Murphy retractor.

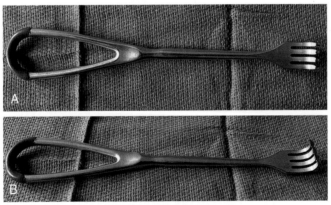

Fig. 2.41 **A** and **B**, Volkman retractor.

Description

A handheld, smooth, flat metal strip with rounded ends (Fig. 2.42). Able to fit the form of the area that is being operated. Various sizes and shapes. It is malleable.

Use(s)

Commonly used in procedures in which organs or intestines need to be retracted.

Instrument Insight

Can be bent or molded as needed

PARKER RETRACTOR[1,2]

Other Names

Park bench retractor, nested right-angle retractor, double round retractor

Category

Retracting and exposing

Description

Double-ended blades with smooth rounded ends (Fig. 2.43).

Use(s)

Used to retract and expose small or shallow wounds.

SKIN HOOK[1,2]

Other Names

Joseph hook, Gillies hook, Freer skin hook, Frazier skin hook

Category

Retracting and exposing

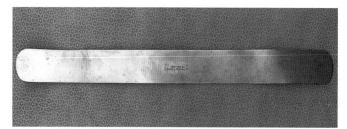

Fig. 2.42 Ribbon retractor.

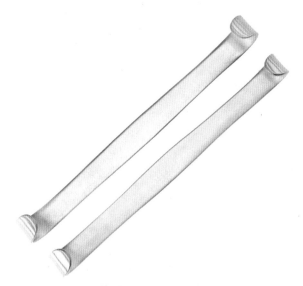

Fig. 2.43 Parker retractor.

Description

Has a sharp hook, with single or double prong. The handle is knurled and round, tapering to the end of the hook (Fig. 2.44).

Use(s)

Lightweight retractors commonly used at the skin edges.

Caution

Hooks are very sharp. Handle the instrument with care and avoid puncture to the glove or skin.

WEITLANER RETRACTOR[1,2]

Category

Retracting and exposing

Description

Instrument shaped like scissors with downward pointing prongs at the tip. Prongs can be either sharp or blunt. There are three prongs on one end and four prongs on the other end. Prongs are all outward curved. The handle includes a ratchet mechanism (Fig. 2.45).

Use(s)

Used to hold tissues, viscera, or skin edges of the incised wound.

GELPI RETRACTOR[1,2]

Category

Retracting and exposing

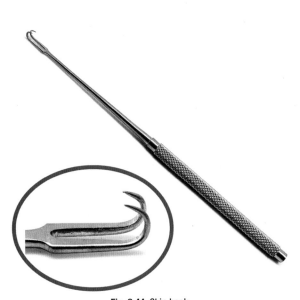

Fig. 2.44 Skin hook.

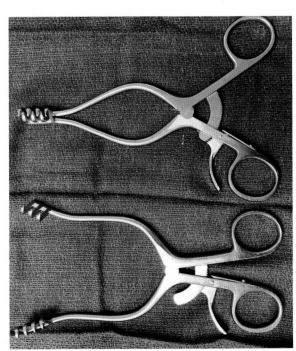

Fig. 2.45 Weitlaner retractor

Description

Has long shanks with two outward-turned sharp prongs, one on each side. Has a locking mechanism to allow the retractor to remain in place (Fig. 2.46).

Use(s)

Used to retract superficial or deep skin layers for better visibility.

FRAZIER SUCTION TIP[1,2]

Category

Suctioning and aspirating

Description

An angled tube with an opening on the handgrip. The diameter of the tube is measured anywhere from 3 to 15 Fr (Fig. 2.47).

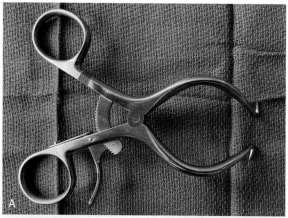

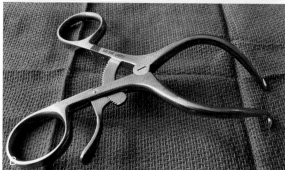

Fig. 2.46 **A** and **B,** Gelpi retractor.

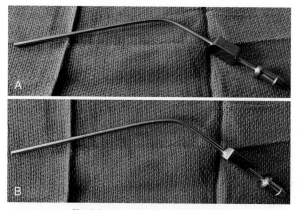

Fig. 2.47 **A** and **B,** Frazier suction tip.

Use(s)

Thin instrument used for removal of fluid or debris from confined surgical spaces.

Instrument Insight

Frazier suction tip also included a thin wire stylet. This is used to push out any debris that may get trapped in the tube while suctioning. The amount of suction is increased by covering the opening on the base of the tip.

YANKAUER SUCTION TIP[1,2]

Other Names

Tonsil suction tip, oral suction tip

Category

Suctioning and aspirating

Description

Firm plastic suction tip with a large opening surrounded by a bulbous head (Fig. 2.48).

Use(s)

Used for suctioning in all types of wounds. Allows for effective suctioning without damage to surrounding tissue.

Instrument Insight

Commonly used to suction oropharyngeal secretion in order to prevent aspirations. Disposable Yankauer is the most widely used suction tip.

CRILE-WOOD NEEDLE HOLDER[1,2]

Other Names

Fine needle holder, Fine needle driver

Category

Suturing and stapling

Description

The blades are less wide and gently taper with a crisscross gripping pattern on the inner jaws with a blunt tip. Has ratcheted finger ring handles. The overall shape and size are very similar to those of a Mayo needle holder, which is more robust in appearance (Fig. 2.49).

Use(s)

Used to hold and guide small- to medium-sized needles and suture material.

MAYO-HEGAR NEEDLE HOLDER[1,2]

Other Name

Heavy needle driver

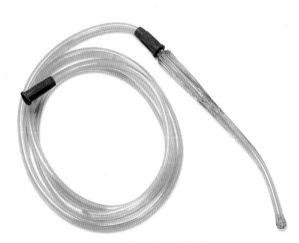

Fig. 2.48 Yankauer suction tip.

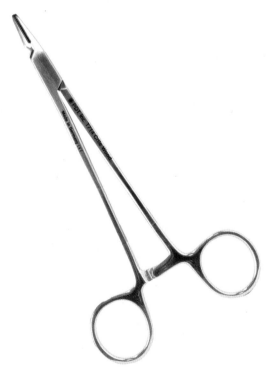

Fig. 2.49 Crile-Wood needle holder.

Category

Suturing and stapling

Description

Crosshatched surface provides a secure grip. Has a broader jaw that is blunt at the tip. The blades do not taper as much as in the case of Crile needle holder. This gives the instrument a robust feel. The tip has a crisscross pattern on the inner jaws (Fig. 2.50).

Use(s)

Designed to hold large suture needles.

DERF NEEDLE HOLDER[1,2]

Other Names

Ryder needle driver, fine needle driver

Category

Suturing and stapling

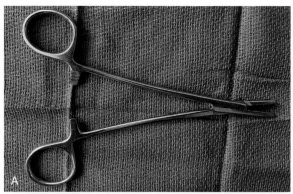
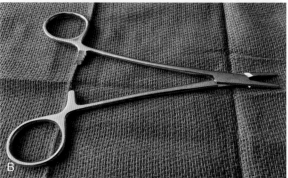

Fig. 2.50 **A** and **B**, Mayo-Hegar needle holder.

Description

It has short, serrated jaws with or without a groove that holds small needles. It is commonly used with 4-0, 5-0, and 6-0 sutures. It is often used to close the skin with 4-0 sutures. Frequently used in ophthalmic, dental, and plastic procedures. The 5-inch length allows it to be easily controlled in smaller surgical areas (Fig. 2.51).

Use(s)

Used for holding delicate to intermediate-sized needles.

Instrument Insight

Commonly used in vascular procedures. Do not use these to grasp large heavy needles.

RYDER NEEDLE HOLDER[1,2]

Other Name

Fine needle holder

Category

Suturing

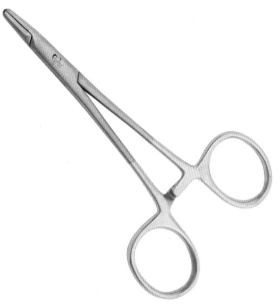

Fig. 2.51 Derf needle holder.

Description

The Ryder needle holder is a ratcheted finger ring instrument that has narrow jaws and is used with very small suture needles in cardiovascular, plastic, and neurosurgical procedures. Its tungsten carbide cross-serrated tips firmly grip the small needle and prevent the needle from twisting or slipping during suturing. This needle holder comes in three different lengths: 6.25, 7.25, and 8.75 inches (Fig. 2.52).

Use(s)

This holder is meant for use with 5-0, 6-0, and 7-0 sized sutures.

NEEDLES[3]

Surgical needles are classified based on the following characteristics.

1. Curve or straight
2. Needle length
3. Cutting or noncutting
4. Regular or reverse cutting
5. Radius
6. Fraction of the curve.

The straight needle is held without any instrument, and suturing is done without a needle holder. This most commonly used to close the last layer of the skin in abdominal incisions (Fig. 2.53).

a. A curved needle is loaded on to a needle holder and is most often used for suturing. It is more precise in closing and aligning the facial planes and can be maneuvered in deep and tighter spaces.

b. Noncutting versus cutting needle: A tapering needle has a cylindrical round shape that tapers to a sharp point at the end. The point helps to make a hole through soft tissue. The rest of the

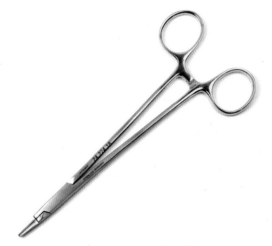

Fig. 2.52 Ryder needle holder.

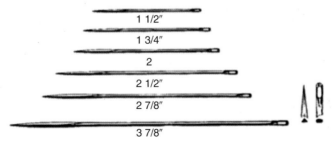

1 1/2"

1 3/4"

2

2 1/2"

2 7/8"

3 7/8"

Fig. 2.53 Straight needles.

needle and suture can easily glide through tissue after the initial cut. The cut created causes minimal trauma to surrounding tissue. After the needle makes its pass, there is good integrity in the tissue that is cut and less risk of tissue being torn when a tight knot is created. The needle is used to suture fascia, muscle, peritoneum, and gut. It is not suitable for skin or tough thick facial layer because the needle will have difficulty going through the tissue (Table 2.1).

c. Conventional cutting versus reverse cutting needle: Regular cutting needles are triangular in shape with the sharp cutting edge on the inside of the needle. Pulling on the needle or lifting the tissue with the needle will cut through surrounding tissue, causing more damage (see Table 2.1).

When tying the knot of the suture, the suture is more likely to pull though the tissue, lacerating it during tying.

The reverse cutting needle has the cutting edge on the outer convex side of the needle. It is less likely to cause damage to surrounding tissue.

SKIN STAPLER[1,2]

Category

Suturing and stapling

Description

Instrument preloaded with stainless steel staples. It includes a handle and a trigger. When the trigger is squeezed, it will place the staple into the skin. There are various different models and manufacturers (Fig. 2.54).

TABLE 2.1 Needle Types and Their Uses	
Needle Type	**Uses**
Taper point	For soft tissues Dilates; does not cut Does not weaken the tissue Good for gastrointestinal, vessel, and soft tissue repair
Reverse cutting	Very sharp Cut through tissue Does not weaken the tissue Good for skin and tough fascia
Conventional cutting	Very sharp Cuts through easily Weakens the tissue Requires more experience to handle it

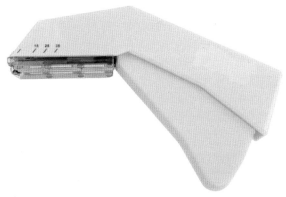

Fig. 2.54 Skin stapler.

Use(s)

Used to close wounds and for skin approximation.

STAPLE REMOVER
Other Name

Staple extractor

Category

Suturing and stapling

Description

The device includes a small upper blunt blade and a lower fenestrated footplate that is thin enough to fit under a staple. The device works by a lever action. When pressure is exerted on handles, the staple bends into an M shape, and the staple is removed from the skin (Fig. 2.55).

Use(s)

Used to remove skin staples from the wound

HEMOCLIP APPLIER[1,2]
Other Names

Clip applier, Wech clip, Ligaclip

Category

Suturing and stapling

Description

It is available in different sizes. The tips are angled and have fine grooves on the inner jaws (Fig. 2.56).

Use(s)

Used for occluding vessels or other tubular structures. The instrument is loaded with clips by the surgical

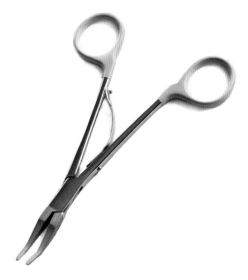

Fig. 2.56 Hemoclip applier.

assistant. A bleeding vessel can be clipped to secure hemostasis.

Conclusion

Instruments are an important part of any surgery. It is very important to be familiar with the them, know their names, and be aware of their appropriate uses. This knowledge will save time in the OR and improve surgical technique. A proceduralist who is clumsy in the OR and is not familiar with the etiquette of handling instruments will not earn respect of his or her team members during procedures. Proper handling of the sharp instruments such as needles and blades is important for everyone's safety in the OR. This will also prevent confusion and any miscounting of instruments, avoiding unnecessary delay at the end of the case.

REFERENCES

1. Nemitz R. Surgical Instrumentation: An Interactive Approach. St Louis: Elsevier; 2019. 3rd ed..
2. Rutherford CJ. Differentiating Surgical Instruments. Philadelphia: FA Davis; 2019.
3. Kreis PG, Fishman SM. Basic surgical skills for the operating room. In: Kries Paul, Fishman Scott, eds. Spinal Cord Stimulation: Percutaneous Implantation Techniques. New York, NY: Oxford University Press; 2009:95–114.

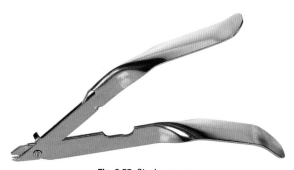

Fig. 2.55 Staple remover.

Chapter 3

Sacroiliac Joint Injection Techniques

Ali Arastu and Tariq Malik

Introduction

The sacroiliac joint (SIJ) is the largest true synovial joint in the body. It is one of the most common sources of chronic low back pain, accounting for 15% to 30% of patients presenting with chronic low back pain.[1] The presentation is variable, physical examination is unreliable, and currently diagnostic injection is the only accepted way to diagnose SIJ pain. The economic burden of chronic SIJ pain is unknown and underappreciated. The quality of life of patients with SIJ pain is worse than that of patients with chronic obstructive pulmonary disease or mild heart failure and is equivalent to that of patients with hip and knee osteoarthritis.[2] Ackerman et al.[3] estimated that pain from degenerative SIJ costs Medicare $18,527 per patient over 5 years. There is no definite treatment or established cure for chronic pain from SIJ. This is because chronic SIJ pain is a syndrome and not one disease. Many structures in and around the SIJ cause or contribute to SIJ pain. History and physical examination are helpful to rule out non-SIJ causes, but current clinical practice relies on a diagnostic SIJ block to properly diagnose SIJ as the pain generator.[4] This chapter discusses the perioperative management of SIJ steroid injections performed under ultrasound and fluoroscopic guidance.

History of Sacroiliac Joint Disorder

From Hippocrates (460–377 BC) to Vaesalius (1514–1564) and until Pare (Vaesalius, 1543; Pare, 1634; Lynch, 1920), the SIJ was considered relevant only during delivery, with no real movement during life, and getting fused or ankylosed with advanced age. It became a focus of interest in the early 20th century, but the landmark study of Mixter and Barr correlating disk rupture with back pain took the focus away from SIJ. The joint injection was described for the first time in 1938, but fluoroscopic guidance was used for the first time in 1979. Better understanding of the joint innervation has led to the innovation of radioablative neurotomy in the 2000s.

The SIJ is a diarthrodial synovial joint between two variably undulating surfaces of the sacrum and ilium, with a capsule strengthened by ligaments. The joint is formed between the S1 to S3 part of the sacrum and the ilium. The articular surfaces are covered with a layer of hyaline cartilage and a superficial layer of fibrocartilage. The combined thickness of the two layers is greater on the sacral side (3 mm) compared with the ilium (0.5 mm). The joint has an auricular or C-shaped, L-shaped configuration with a short cranial and a longer caudal limb. The sacral part is generally concave often with an intraarticular bony tubercle present in the middle aspect of the auricular surface of the sacrum. The iliac part is reciprocally convex. The caudal limb of this C- or L-shaped joint is the synovial aspect of the joint, and the upper part of the cranial limb is the fibrous joint.

The joint has very limited movement. In bipedal gait, the joint is a relay station of forces from the upper body down the legs and vice versa. It moves in all three axes. The mobility depends on positioning and the distribution of load but is usually limited to 2 degrees. The joint can rotate and glide up and down, as well as back and forth, but rotation of the sacrum (nutation and counternutation) around its transverse axis at S2 is considered to be the main movement.

The joint is well innervated, but details are not well known. Innervation from the ventral lumbosacral rami is reported but not verified, but innervations from the dorsal rami are well accepted. Contributions from L5 to S3 are reported, which include branches from the superior gluteal nerve, dorsal and ventral rami, and obturator nerve. Grob et al.[5] argued that the SIJ is chiefly innervated by the dorsal sacral rami, based on their finding that all the nerve fibers identified by fetal dissection came from the dorsal mesenchyme.

Indications

Patients suspected of having SIJ pain are selected for joint injection. Even though the predictive value of clinical features (history and physical examination) is limited, it is a good starting point.[6] Pain is mechanical in nature, with pain felt in the buttock or back of the thigh. Classically, SIJ pain is often reported as pain below L5. There are a number of clinical examination maneuvers, such as the FABER (flexion, abduction and external rotation) test, the Gaenslen test, the Gillet test, Yoeman's test, the distraction test, and various compression tests, that can elicit pain stemming from SIJ dysfunction. They are provocation tests designed to elicit pain by stressing the joint. If at least three of these provocative maneuvers elicit pain, the patient is clinically suspected to have pain originating from the SIJ.[7] This can be confirmed with a diagnostic SIJ block. Imaging of the spine, pelvis, or both is done to exclude other causes. Magnetic resonance imaging (MRI) is more useful than computed tomography in excluding inflammatory and neoplastic causes. MRI of the pelvis with a focus on the sacrum is also useful in diagnosing stress fractures of the sacrum, an important uncommon but underappreciated cause of chronic low back pain that mimics SIJ pain.[8] Current literature states a subjective reported score greater than 75% acute relief of pain after injection is diagnostic of an SIJ source of pain.[9]

Patient Selection

Patients are selected for injection therapy (diagnostic or therapeutic) if
1. Clinical features are suggestive of SIJ pain.
2. Other causes of pain have been excluded.
3. Pain is chronic (at least 3 months).
4. Pain is intense (>5/10) or affecting quality of life.

5. The patient has failed conservative therapy (e.g., physical therapy, nonsteroidal antiinflammatory drugs).
6. There are no contraindications to injection therapy.

Contraindications

Absolute contraindications include:
1. Inability or refusal to give consent

Relative contraindications include:
1. Patient-reported or documented history of allergic reaction to cortisone injections
2. Local malignancy
3. Coagulopathy or current or recent use of blood-thinning agents
4. Pregnancy
5. Systemic infection, septic joint, or osteomyelitis
6. Type 2 diabetes with a history of poor glycemic control[8]

Preprocedure Considerations

Preprocedure considerations for SIJ injections are similar to those for most outpatient pain procedures. The procedure itself is low risk and not very painful. The medication and the needle used in the procedure pose no major risk to the patient. The joint has no vital structure around it that can pose a major risk. The main risk of the injection is patient dependent. The patient's habitus and the underlying medical conditions may make the injection challenging. Important preprocedure considerations are
1. Evaluate major comorbidities. The procedure is elective. The patient should be in optimal medical condition if possible. Optimal metabolic (e.g., blood sugar) and cardiovascular management is desirable.
2. Review medications, especially anticoagulants, and whether they need to be discontinued or not. In general, most medications can be continued. The American Society of Regional Anesthesia app is very helpful.
3. Have appropriate laboratory testing performed if needed.
4. If sedation is planned for the procedure, then appropriate instruction should be given regarding

NPO (nothing by mouth) status, a ride home, and so on.

5. Have a pregnancy test performed if fluoroscopy is used and if the test is indicated.
6. Review drug allergies carefully, especially to radiocontrast dye.
7. Provide intravenous access if needed for anxiolysis or potential drug reaction.
8. Evaluate the patient's ability to lie in a prone position. It is a short procedure, but many patients may not be able to stay still for 10 to 15 minutes because of their body habitus or other painful parts of the body. This is especially an issue when trainees are doing the procedure under supervision because of the extended time needed.
9. Document lower extremity strength because there is a potential for lower extremity weakness from the injectate.

Attention to the multitude of factors involved in caring for these patients is essential to decrease morbidity from this procedure.

Equipment and Supplies

1. C-arm and table
2. Procedure tray
3. Sterile drape
4. Antiseptic scrub (alcohol, povidone-iodine, and chlorhexidine)
5. Quincke spinal needle: 22 or 25 gauge × 3.5 inches
6. 25-gauge, 1-inch needle for skin infiltration
7. Syringes
   a. Two 3-mL syringes
   b. One 5-mL syringe
8. J-loop or short extension tubing
9. Sterile gauze
10. Adhesive bandages
11. Local anesthetic
    a. 1% to 2% lidocaine for the skin wheal
    b. Bupivacaine 0.25% to 0.5% for the joint
    c. Steroids (any of the following)
       (1) Triamcinolone acetate
       (2) Betamethasone
       (3) Dexamethasone
12. Injectate
    a. Diagnostic injection: bupivacaine

b. Therapeutic injection: bupivacaine and steroid

The volume of the injectate is kept at 2 mL or less because the joint volume in anatomic studies has shown that the mean joint volume is 1.08 mL (range, 1–2.5 mL).

Step-by-Step Image-Guided Technique

Although SIJ injections can be performed without imaging guidance, according to various studies, there is only a 12% to 22% chance of the needle reaching the SIJ with a landmark technique.[7] This portion of the text explains the step-by-step guide of SIJ injections with fluoroscopic guidance. The technique was described by Dr. Dussault originally in 2000.[10]

STEP-BY-STEP GUIDE
Fluoroscopic-Guided Approach

1. Confirmed documentation of consent. A time out should be done: correct patient, correct procedure, and correct laterality.
2. Have the patient lie prone on the procedure table (Fig. 3.1).

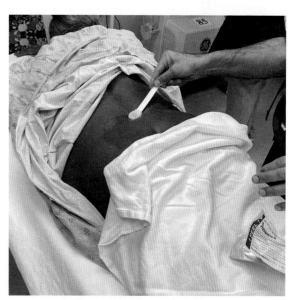

Fig. 3.1 A patient prone on the table.

3. Prep and drape the patient's low back and gluteal area (Fig. 3.2).
4. Draw lidocaine for the skin in a 3-mL syringe, radiopaque dye in a 5-mL syringe, and the injectate in a 3-mL syringe.
5. All medications are labeled to avoid any drug error.
6. Take an anteroposterior view of the joint (Fig. 3.3).
7. Tilt the C-arm 20 to 25 degrees, with the image intensifier above the patient, in the cephalad direction, toward the patient's head. This moves the anterior part of the joint out of the way, exposing the posterior accessible part of the joint.
8. The C-arm is tilted in a contralateral direction at 5 to 20 degrees to fine tune the outline of the inferior part of the joint by superimposing SIJ lines (Fig. 3.4).
9. The target is the inferiormost part of the joint. The goal is to be 1 to 2 cm above the inferior end of the joint (Fig. 3.5).
10. The skin entry point is numbed using 25-gauge needle using 1% to 2% lidocaine, and a

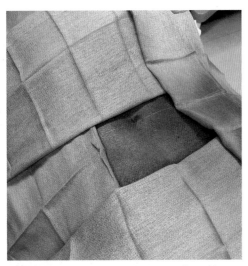

Fig. 3.2 The area draped with blue sterile towels.

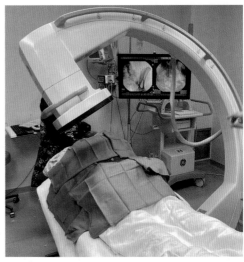

Fig. 3.4 The C-arm tilted in a contralateral direction to outline the sacroiliac joint.

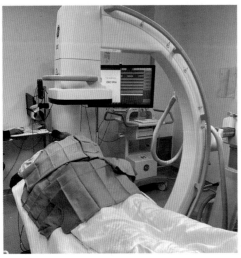

Fig. 3.3 Anteroposterior view of the sacroiliac joint.

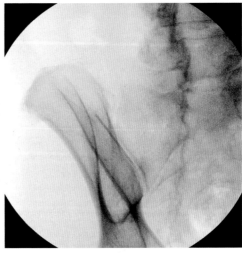

Fig. 3.5 The needle pointing to sacroiliac joint entry point.

22-gauge spinal needle is advanced under fluoroscopic guidance using a bull's eye approach (Figs. 3.6 and 3.7).

11. Minimize radiation exposure to the patient and others in the procedure room by observing the principles of ALARA (as low as reasonably achievable).

12. When the needle tip pierces the capsule or ligament, it may reproduce the patient's back pain.

13. The needle should be advanced a few millimeters until it is well within the joint. Angling laterally helps because this is the natural curvature of the joint.

14. The depth of the needle should be confirmed in the lateral view to ensure the needle has not advanced in front of the sacrum (Fig. 3.8).

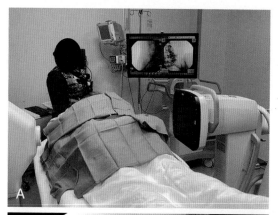

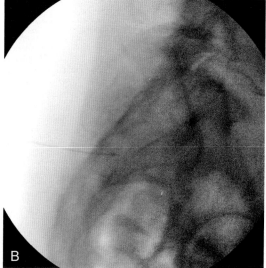

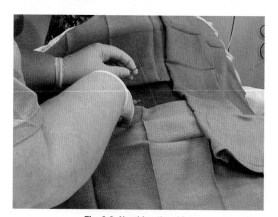

Fig. 3.6 Numbing the skin.

Fig. 3.8 **A,** Lateral view of the needle. **B,** Properly placed needle-tip will be ventral to the Sacrum.

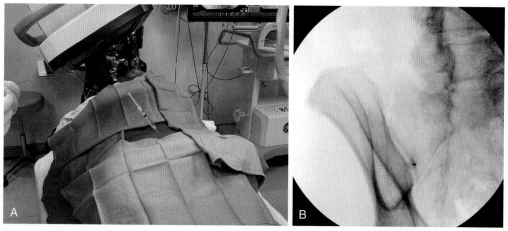

Fig. 3.7 **A,** Skin and tissue along the x-ray beam. **B,** Needle advanced inplane towards the joint.

15. Inject 0.5 mL of the contrast solution to confirm proper placement (Fig. 3.9).
16. After the proper needle tip placement is confirmed by intraarticular spread of the contrast, then inject 2.0 mL of the injectate (local anesthetic with or without steroid) (Fig. 3.10).
17. Pull the needle out of the joint and flush any steroid out of the needle before removing the needle all the way out of the body to avoid tracking steroid to the skin, which can cause hypopigmentation.
18. Apply a bandage to cover the skin puncture site.

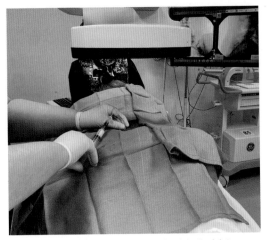

Fig. 3.10 Injecting steroid solution into the joint.

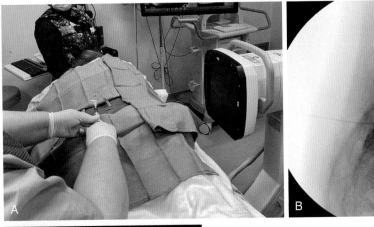

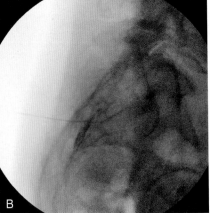

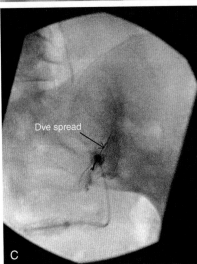

Dye spread

Fig. 3.9 A and **B**, Injection of dye confirming intracapsular needle position. **C**, Anteroposterior image of sacroiliac joint revealing intraarticular spread of dye.

Ultrasound-Guided Approach

The injection can be performed with ultrasound guidance instead of fluoroscopy.

Position: The patient is placed in a prone position (Fig. 3.11).

Probe: C-50 (low-frequency curvilinear probe).

Supplies: The same in addition to ultrasound probe cover and gel.

Steps:

1. The probe is place horizontally over the sacral cornu, just cranial to the coccyx, seen as a single bony outline in the middle of the screen (Fig. 3.12).
2. The probe is slid laterally to visualize the second bony outline of the ilium (Fig. 3.13).

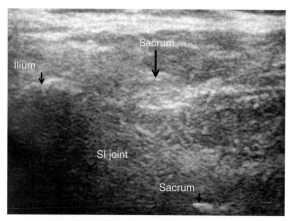

Fig. 3.13 Ultrasound view of the sacroiliac joint.

3. The probe is moved cranially until the cleft between the ileum and sacrum is seen. This is usually at the level of the S2 foramen.
4. It is important to keep an eye on the sacral foramina as hypoechoic gaps within the outline of the sacrum.
5. The three prominent pointy outlines can be seen in the dorsal outline of the sacrum; these are the median crest, medial crest, and lateral crest. The medial crest and lateral crest are on either side of the sacral foramina.
6. After identifying the cleft between the sacrum and ileum, a 22-gauge spinal needle is advanced in an in-plane medial-to-lateral direction (Fig. 3.14).

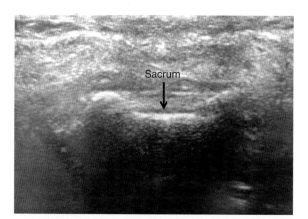

Fig. 3.11 The patient is placed prone, and the area is draped.

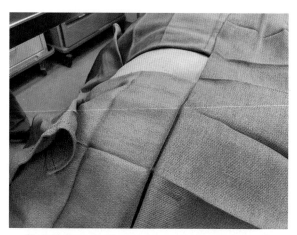

Fig. 3.12 Ultrasound view with the probe placed over the sacrum.

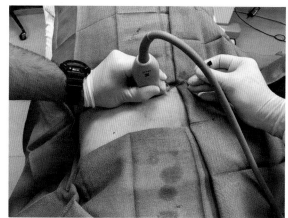

Fig. 3.14 In-plane ultrasound view of sacroiliac joint injection.

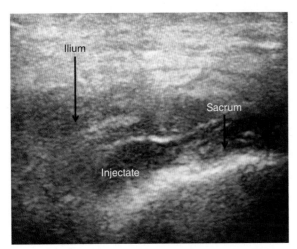

Fig. 3.15 Ultrasound view shows injectate confined within the joint.

7. When the needle is in the joint, 2 to 3 mL of the solution is injected.
8. Proper needle tip position is confirmed by visualizing the tip and spread of solution. The needle should be close to the cleft, with minimal fluid escaping the joint (Fig. 3.15).
9. Ultrasound guidance is helpful in patients with allergy to iodine or seafood because it obviates the need to use the contrast.

Ultrasound-guided and fluoroscopically guided SIJ injections have been compared in two randomized controlled trials. In a study by Jee et al.,[11] ultrasonography provided lower accuracy than fluoroscopy (87.3% vs 98.2%, respectively), Soneji et al.[12] found a lower, but not statistically significant, difference in the incidence of intraarticular spread in the ultrasound group versus the fluoroscopic group (50% vs 65%, respectively) with similar improvement on follow-up.

REGENERATIVE INJECTION THERAPY

Sacroiliac joint injection with steroids is the most commonly used medication that is effective against SIJ pain. Because of its short-term effects, other modalities such as platelet-rich plasma (PRP) or mesenchymal stem cells (MSCs) can be considered when performing SIJ injections. PRP is an autologous biological blood-derived product that can be exogenously applied to various tissues wherein it releases high concentrations of platelet-derived growth factors that enhance the body's natural healing response.[13] When comparing PRP with steroid injections, PRP showed 90% patient-reported satisfactory relief compared with 25% relief in patients receiving steroids at a 3-month follow-up visit.[14] MSCs are cells that can differentiate into almost any end-stage lineage cells based on the scaffold they are seeded to.[15] This property makes them an ideal source for tissue regeneration and tissue healing. For MSC injections, Sanapati et al. have shown improved pain relief in patients with discogenic pain, although there are few data for its use in SIJ injections.

LEVEL OF EVIDENCE

Sacroiliac joint injection therapy for the management of chronic refractory pain has been reviewed extensively with the conclusion that quality of evidence for the intraarticular and a periarticular steroid injection is limited to poor.[16]

Postprocedure Considerations

After completion of the SIJ injection, patients are taken to a postoperative room for observation. Basic vital signs are checked. The injection site is checked to ensure there is no swelling (from bleeding). More important, the lower extremities are examined for any motor weakness. SIJ injections are generally safe procedures. Most commonly described side effects include pain, vasovagal reaction, facial flushing or sweating, and transient sciatic nerve block (from anterior capsular disruption) with associated fall risk.[17,18] Rarer, but more serious, complications include trauma to the nerves, accidental intervertebral foraminal injection (injuring pelvic structure if fluoroscopic guidance is improper), hematoma formation, sciatic palsy, meningitis, abscess, and systemic infection. There have also been a reported case of pyogenic sacroiliitis and a case of herpes simplex.[19] Providers should also be cautious of the possibility of systemic steroid absorption. Adverse effects include hyperglycemia, decreased bone mineral density with possible increased fracture risk, immunosuppression with increased risk of infection, Cushing syndrome, and hypothalamic–pituitary axis suppression.[17]

Management if Failed

A technical unsuccessful rate of 10% has been reported by multiple studies.[20] Patients who fail to achieve initial relief after SIJ injection with anesthetic and steroid are very unlikely to achieve significant pain relief at follow-up.[21] If failed, patients can choose to try the SIJ injection again later. Otherwise, other interventions may be considered, including prolotherapy, radiofrequency ablation, viscosupplementation, or minimally invasive SIJ fusion.[20] Providers should also think of other causes of pain.[22] The differential diagnosis consists of myofascial pain, trochanteric bursitis, piriformis syndrome, cluneal nerve entrapment, lumbosacral disk herniation or bulge, lumbosacral facet syndrome, and lumbar radiculopathy.[23]

REFERENCES

1. Chuang CW, Hung SK, Pan PT, Kao MC. Diagnosis and interventional pain management options for sacroiliac joint pain. *Ci Ji Yi Xue Za Zhi.* 2019;31(4):207-210.
2. Owen DS. Aspiration and injection of joints and soft tissues. In: Kelley WN, ed. *Textbook of Rheumatology.* 5th ed. Philadelphia: Saunders; 1997:591-608.
3. Ackerman SJ, Polly DW, Knight T. Nonoperative care to manage sacroiliac joint disruption and degenerative sacroiliitis: high costs and medical resource utilization in the United States Medicare population. *J Neurosurg Spine.* 2014;20:354-356.
4. Mitchell B, MacPhail T, Vivian D, Verrills P, Barnard A. Diagnostic sacroiliac joint injections: us a control block necessary [abstract]? *J Sci Med Sport.* 2015;12(suppl 2):e5-e6.
5. Grob KR, Neuhuber WL, Kissling RO. Innervation of the sacroiliac joint of the human. *Z Rheumatol.* 1995;54(2):117–122.
6. Bernard Jr TN, Kirkaldy-Willis WH. Recognizing specific characteristics of nonspecific low back pain. *Clin Orthop Relat Res.* 1987;(217):266-280.
7. Ackerman SJ, Polly DW, Knight T. Nonoperative care to manage sacroiliac joint disruption and degenerative sacroiliitis: high costs and medical resource utilization in the United States Medicare population. *J Neurosurg Spine.* 2014;20:354-356.
8. Raj MA, Ampat G, Varacallo M. Sacroiliac Joint Pain. [Updated 2022 Sep 4]. In: StatPearls [Internet]. Treasure Island (FL): StatPearls Publishing; 2022 Jan-. Available from: https://www.ncbi.nlm.nih.gov/books/NBK470299/
9. Cher D, Polly D, Berven S. Sacroiliac joint pain: burden of disease. *Med Devices (Auckl).* 2014;7:73-81.
10. Dussault RG, Kaplan PA, Anderson NW. Fluoroscopy-guided sacroiliac joint injections. *Radiology.* 2000;214(1):273-277.
11. Jee Haemi, Lee Ji-Hae, Park Ki Deok, Ahn Jaeki, Park Yongbum. Ultrasound-guided versus fluoroscopy-guided sacroiliac joint intra-articular injections in the noninflammatory sacroiliac joint dysfunction: a prospective, randomized, single-blinded study. *Arch Phys Med Rehabil.* 2014;95(2):330–337. doi:10.1016/j.apmr.2013.09.021.
12. Soneji Neilesh, Bhatia Anuj, Seib Rachael, Tumber Paul, Dissanayake Melanie, Peng Philip WH. Comparison of fluoroscopy and ultrasound guidance for sacroiliac joint injection in patients with chronic low back pain. *Pain Pract.* 2016;16(5):537–544. doi:10.1111/papr.12304.
13. Wroblewski AP, Mejia HA, Wright VJ. Application of platelet-rich plasma to enhance tissue repair. *Oper Tech Orthop.* 2010;20:98-105.
14. Singla V, Batra YK, Bharti N, et al. Steroid vs. platelet-rich plasma in ultrasound-guided sacroiliac joint injection for chronic low back pain. *Pain Pract.* 2017;17(6):782-791.
15. Han Y, Li X, Zhang Y, Han Y, Chang F, Ding J. Mesenchymal stem cells for regenerative medicine. *Cells.* 2019;8(8):886.
16. Sanapati J, Manchikanti L, Atluri S, et al. Do regenerative medicine therapies provide long-term relief in chronic low back pain: a systematic review and metaanalysis. *Pain Physician.* 2018;21(6):515-540.
17. Zheng P, Schneider BJ, Yang A, McCormick ZL. Image-guided sacroiliac joint injections: an evidence-based review of best practices and clinical outcomes. *PM R.* 2019;11(suppl 1):S98-S104.
18. Kennedy DJ, Schneider B, Casey E, et al. Vasovagal rates in fluoroscopically guided interventional procedures: a study of over 8,000 injections. *Pain Med.* 2013;14(12):1854-1859.
19. Plastaras CT, Joshi AB, Garvan C, et al. Adverse events associated with fluoroscopically guided sacroiliac joint injections. *PM R.* 2012;4(7):473-478.
20. Wu L, Tafti D, Varacallo M. Sacroiliac Joint Injection. [Updated 2022 Sep 7]. In: StatPearls [Internet]. Treasure Island (FL): StatPearls Publishing; 2022. Available at: https://www.ncbi.nlm.nih.gov/books/NBK513245/.
21. Schneider BJ, Huynh L, Levin J, et al. Does immediate pain relief after an injection into the sacroiliac joint with anesthetic and corticosteroid predict subsequent pain relief? *Pain Med.* 2018;19(2):244-251.
22. Le Huec JC, Tsoupras A, Leglise A, Heraudet P, Celarier G, Sturresson B. The Sacro-Iliac joint: a potentially painful enigma. Update on the diagnosis and treatment of pain from microtrauma. *Orthop Traumatol Surg Res.* 2019;105(suppl 1):S31-S42.
23. Schmidt GL, Bhandutia AK, Altman DT. Management of sacroiliac joint pain. *J Am Acad Orthop Surg.* 2018;26(17):610-616.

Chapter 4

Sacral Lateral Branch Nerve Block

Evan Parker, Christine Zaky, and George Girgis

Introduction

Sacroiliac joint (SIJ) pain is one of the most common causes of axial low back pain. Studies have shown that 13% to 30% of chronic axial low back pain is related to the SIJ.[1] This wide variability of reporting is related to the methodology used to confirm the diagnosis. Innervation of the SIJ is variable with most literature reporting S1 to S3 lateral branches as the main nerve supply with contribution from the L5 dorsal ramus and possible innervation from the L4 medial branch and S4 lateral branch (Fig. 4.1). Administration of local anesthetic to the L5 dorsal ramus and the lateral branches of S1 to S3 has been described as a diagnostic tool before denervation of the SIJ. These blocks have a predictive value for positive outcomes after radiofrequency ablation (RFA) for treatment of patients with chronic SIJ pain.[2]

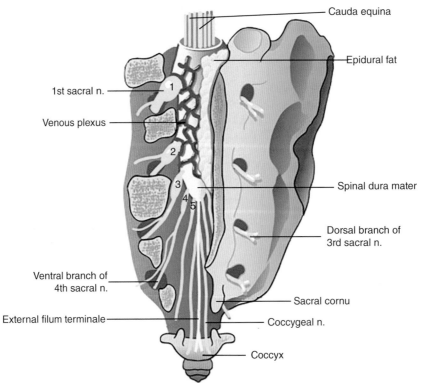

Fig. 4.1 Anatomy of the sacral spine region. *n,* Nerve. (From Waldman SD. *Atlas of Interventional Pain Management.* 4th ed. Philadelphia: Saunders; 2015:578.)

Indications

Sacral lateral branch nerve block is usually done as a diagnostic test before denervation of the SIJs for long-term pain relief. It has a more predictive value for favorable outcomes after RFA than intraarticular or periarticular injection.[3-5]

Contraindications

Contraindications to the diagnostic sacroiliac joint, sacral lateral branches nerve block:
- Systemic or local site infection
- Anticoagulation (relative)
- Allergy to medications
- Patient refusal

Diagnosis

The diagnosis depends mainly on history and physical examination. Patients commonly report pain with transitional activities such as rising from a seated position or getting out of bed. Pain is described as unilateral or bilateral pain below the belt line with occasional radiation along posterior thigh to the ipsilateral knee (pseudo-radiculopathy). International Association for the Study of Pain diagnostic criteria[6] include a positive Fortin finger test result (pain within 1 cm inferior-medial to the posterior superior iliac spine), three or more positive provocative test results (Faber, Gaenslen, compression, distraction, and so on), and pain that is relieved by injection of the SIJ with the latter reported to be the most specific tool.

Radiologic findings can help confirm the diagnosis and vary from SIJ sclerosis to significant degenerative changes.[7]

Procedure

The patient is positioned in the prone position with a C-arm in either an anteroposterior (AP) or with a slight cephalocaudal angle to optimize appearance of sacral foramina. The patient's legs and heels are abducted to prevent tightening of the gluteal muscles, which can obscure the view of the sacrum. A wide prep is then completed with an antiseptic solution. Lidocaine 1% is then used to anesthetize the skin. A 22- or 25-gauge spinal needle is advanced under fluoroscopic guidance to the location of the ipsilateral L5 dorsal ramus using the AP and oblique views (L4 could be completed if desired; Fig. 4.2). The 22- or 25-gauge spinal needles are then advanced to a point approximately 5 mm lateral to the ipsilateral S1, S2, and S3 sacral foramina, corresponding to the pathway of the lateral branch

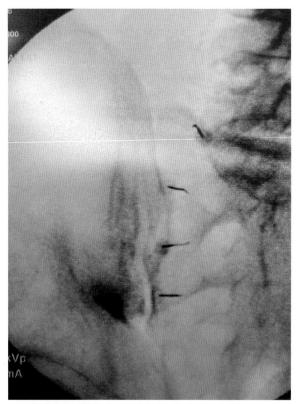

Fig. 4.2 Anteroposterior view showing needles positioned lateral to the S1 to S3 foramen and close to the L5 dorsal ramus.

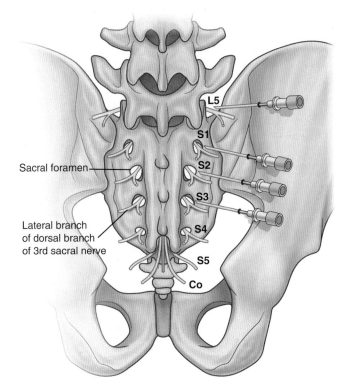

Sacral foramen

Lateral branch
of dorsal branch
of 3rd sacral nerve

L5
S1
S2
S3
S4
S5
Co

Fig. 4.3 Correct anatomic needle placement for lateral branches of S1, S2, and S3 nerve root block.

nerves at S1 to S3 (Fig. 4.3). After the position of the needles is confirmed, a lateral fluoroscopic view is obtained to ensure adequate depth. After negative aspiration of blood and cerebrospinal fluid, 0.5 mL of 0.5% bupivacaine is injected at each level.

The patient is then instructed to monitor pain and record their pain scores every 30 minutes for 8 hours. About 60% to 80% improvement in pain scores for 4 to 8 hours after this block is considered a positive outcome predicting RFA success.

Potential Complications

Like any other procedures, potential complications could develop in relation to the technique, anatomic site, radiation exposure, or medications injected.
- Infection and bleeding are rare.
- Intravascular injection: Local anesthetic systemic toxicity (LAST) is a rare event because the volume injected for this block is minimal.

- Intrathecal injection could result in transient motor weakness.
- Nerve damage to sacral nerve roots may occur.
- Radiation exposure complications may occur.
- Medication-related complications could develop from a minor allergic reaction to an extreme anaphylactic shock.

REFERENCES

1. Cheng J, Chen SL, Zimmerman N, Dalton JE, LaSalle G, Rosenquist R. A new radiofrequency ablation procedure to treat sacroiliac joint pain. *Pain Physician.* 2016;19(8):603-615.
2. Cohen SP, Abdi S. Lateral branch blocks as a treatment for sacroiliac joint pain: a pilot study. *Reg Anesth Pain Med.* 2003;28(2): 113-119.
3. Dreyfuss P, Henning T, Malladi N, Goldstein B, Bogduk N. The ability of multi-site, multi-depth sacral lateral branch blocks to anesthetize the sacroiliac joint complex. *Pain Med.* 2009;10(4): 679-688.
4. Cohen SP, Hurley RW, Buckenmaier CC III, et al. Randomized placebo-controlled study evaluating lateral branch radiofrequency

denervation for sacroiliac joint pain. *Anesthesiology*. 2008;109(2):279-288.

5. Luukkainen RK, Wennerstrand PV, Kautiainen HH, Sanila MT, Asikainen EL. Efficacy of periarticular corticosteroid treatment of the sacroiliac joint in non-spondylarthropathic patients with chronic low back pain in the region of the sacroiliac joint. *Clin Exp Rheumatol*. 2002;20(1):52.

6. Merskey H, Bogduk N. *Classification of Chronic Pain: Descriptions of Chronic Pain Syndromes and Definitions of Pain Terms*. Seattle, WA: IASP Press; 1994:190-191.

7. O'Shea FD, Boyle E, Salonen DC, et al. Inflammatory and degenerative sacroiliac joint disease in primary back pain cohort. *Arthritis Care Res (Hoboken)*. 2010;62(4):447-454.

Chapter 5

Sacroiliac Joint Radiofrequency Ablation

Timothy J. Woodin, Nasir Hussain, and Alaa Abd-Elsayed

Introduction

Low back pain remains one of the most debilitating and prevalent symptoms in the United States, with a lifetime prevalence of 65% to 70%.[1] The sacroiliac joint (SIJ) is one of the most common causes of chronic low back pain and is found to be the source in 15% to 30% of cases.[2] As the largest synovial joint in the body, the SIJ remains a difficult location, anatomically, to treat back pain given its location in the pelvis. The SIJ connects the sacrum and the ilium and is centrally located adjacent to many motor and sensory nerves of the lower extremities. It has multiple ligaments and stabilizing muscles that keep the joint stable and allow the pelvis to carry the entire weight of the torso. Multiple causes of SIJ pain exist, and there exist several strategies to target this joint.[3] Radiofrequency ablation (RFA) of the SIJ is one such approach that has recently started to gain traction. This chapter briefly reviews the causes of SIJ pain and dives deeper into the therapeutic approaches to SIJ RFA, as well as the relevant anatomy, indications for therapy, contraindications, and complications of the procedure.

Causes of Sacroiliac Joint Pain

Before a discussion regarding RFA of the SIJ, an understanding of the common causes is needed, which has also been presented in detail in prior chapters. Briefly, traumatic causes of SIJ pain are typically due to mechanisms that create strong shearing and rotational forces on the hips. These are typically caused by falls, motor vehicle accidents, or major pelvic trauma. In contrast, multiple atraumatic causes of SIJ pain exist, including osteoarthritis, rheumatoid arthritis, ankylosing spondylitis, inflammatory bowel disease (IBD), and pregnancy. Osteoarthritis typically occurs in adults toward the fifth and sixth decades of life and presents with chronic low back pain with no clear or definite mechanism of injury or traumatic event. Rheumatoid arthritis has a similar picture clinically and symptomology is typically identical to that of osteoarthritis; however, the patient will have more systemic sequalae of their rheumatoid arthritis. Ankylosing spondylitis is a spondylarthritis with axial involvement and is characterized by enthesitis (pain at ligament–tendon insertion points). Other inflammatory states, including IBD, such as Crohn's disease and ulcerative colitis, can present with bilateral SI pathology, and a portion of these patients carry the HLA-B27 antigen. Pregnancy has multiple effects on the SIJ, including laxity and movement of the joint. This can change the loading and stressing forces on the joint space and the entire pelvis and commonly results in pain.

Anatomic Considerations

The SIJ is centrally located joint that connects the sacrum and the ilium bilaterally and has anterior and posterior components. The SIJ is a synovial joint that is stabilized by multiple ligaments and muscles, including the piriformis, gluteus

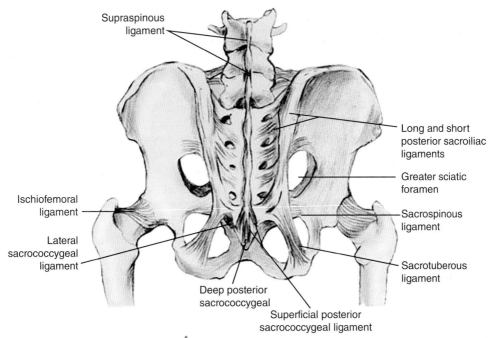

Fig. 5.1 **The sacroiliac joint with associated ligaments.** (Source: Benzon HT, Rathmell JP, Wu CL, Turk DC, et al. *Practical Management of Pain*. 5th ed. St. Louis: Elsevier; 2014.)

maximus, and biceps femoris (Fig. 5.1). The posterior two-thirds of the joint include multiple complex ligamentous attachments that help limit the amount of mobility and the effects of weight changes and shearing forces.[4] SIJ innervation can vary greatly and is typically debated by multiple experts. The posterior segment is typically innervated by the S1 to S3 dorsal rami, as well as the L5 dorsal ramus.[5] In contrast, the anterior joint is typically thought to be supplied by the L2 to S2 ventral rami; however, some believe that there is no specific innervation for the anterior segment.

Patient Selection and Indications

The primary indication for RFA therapy is diagnosing SIJ pain that is refractory to conservative therapies. The most specific test for diagnosing intraarticular SIJ pain is the intraarticular diagnostic block, which should be done before any RFA.[6] This is done via image-guided injection of local anesthetic into the synovial SIJ. The two most common types of SIJ steroid injections and diagnostic nerve blocks are at the

L4 to L5 dorsal rami or S1 to S3 lateral branches. After two consecutive blocks that provide more than 50% relief of a patient's pain symptoms, it can be concluded that a patient is a good candidate for RFA.[7]

Contraindications

Contraindications to any intervention apply in these cases as well. These include overlying skin infection; significant coagulopathies, which increase bleeding risk; and allergies, which prevent the procedure from occurring. Also, most procedures rely on the patient to provide feedback regarding stimulation and sensation (i.e., radicular pain and muscle weakness); therefore, any condition that prevents the patient from being fully alert, awake, and engaged puts the success of the procedure at risk.

Step-by-Step Guide

Sacroiliac joint RFA is a relatively new intervention, with the first occurrence reported in 2001, when 36%

of patients had pain reduction by at least 50% as a result of the procedure.[5] Since then, RFA has become increasingly popular, and advancements have been made, resulting in more effective and safer interventions. However, data still remain sparse and is growing.[8] In its entirety, SIJ RFA aims to destroy nerve endings that transmit pain from the SIJ, therefore relieving pain. Although the innervation of the SIJ varies, most practitioners target the L4 medial branch nerve, L5 dorsal ramus, or S4 lateral branch nerve.[9] RFA is achieved by inserting a probe at the location of the nerve ending and applying electrical current, which then produces a thermal effect thereby lesioning the nerve. There are three common techniques that are used for RFA: Simplicity, strip lesioning, and radiofrequency lesioning. These are discussed in the detail next.

SIMPLICITY

The Simplicity needle was created by Abbott specifically for RFA of the SIJ. Traditional techniques require multiple needle placements for either bipolar or cooled RFA; however, Simplicity requires a single insertion point with a specialized probe that creates five separate lesions to ablate the L5 dorsal ramus and the S1 to S4 lateral branches at a single time (Figs. 5.2 and 5.3). Like traditional RFA, the Simplicity is done under fluoroscopy guidance with a team consisting of the physician, radiology technician, and support staff. The room should be fitted with an

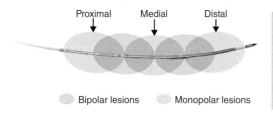

Heating sequence:

1. A bipolar lesion is made between the distal and medial electrodes.
2. A bipolar lesionn is made between the medial and proximal electrodes.
3. A monopolar lesion is made at the distal electrode.
4. A monopolar lesion is made at the medial electrode.
5. A monopolar lesion is made at the proximal electrode.

Fig. 5.2 Simplicity radiofrequency ablation probe creating five lesions with a single insertion point. (Reproduced with permission of Abbott, © 2022. All rights reserved.)

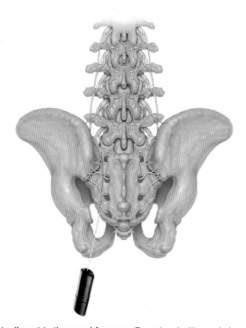

Fig. 5.3 Simplicity probe placement adjacent to the sacral foramen. (Reproduced with permission of Abbott, © 2022. All rights reserved.)

adjustable surgical table and a mobile C-arm (Fig. 5.4). First, the patient is placed in the prone position on the table with padding or a pillow beneath their abdomen to reduce lordosis of the spine. Next, the grounding pad is placed on a muscular area of the body near the procedure site, with care to avoid any hair, bony prominences, significant scars, and any location where fluids may accumulate. Next, the patient's lower back and buttocks are sterilely prepped and draped at the treatment site. Using the C-arm, an anteroposterior (AP) image with the ipsilateral sacrum in view is obtained. This view allows one to identify the insertion point, which is typically 1 cm lateral and inferior to the S4 foramen (see Fig. 5.4). Next a 25-gauge spinal needle and local anesthetic (with or without corticosteroid) is used to anesthetize the track that the Simplicity probe will take when performing the RFA. The spinal needle is advanced just lateral to S4 foramen in a cephalad fashion to the sacral foramen and then advanced through the ligaments between the sacrum and ileum (Fig. 5.5). After withdrawing the stylet from the spinal needle, local anesthetic is injected while the entire needle is

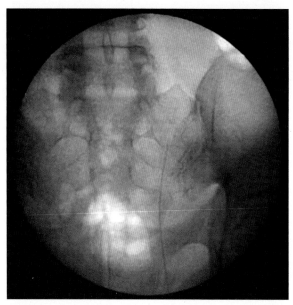

Fig. 5.5 Course of spinal needle while anesthetizing for Simplicity radiofrequency ablation. (Reproduced with permission of Abbott, © 2022. All rights reserved.)

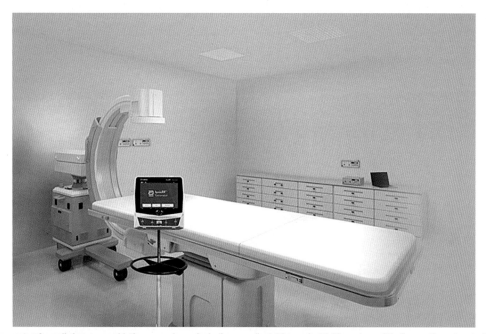

Fig. 5.4 Room setup for radiofrequency ablation procedures, including an adjustable surgical table and a mobile C-arm. (Reproduced with permission of Abbott, © 2022. All rights reserved.)

removed to anesthetize the track. Next, the Simplicity probe is inserted at the original spinal needle entry site. Of note, a small scalpel incision may be necessary to facilitate probe insertion. While advancing the Simplicity probe, lateral images may need to be obtained to ensure lack of probe entry into any of the sacral foramen. The Simplicity probe should then be advanced until contact is made with the sacral ala under AP view, and lateral images should be used to confirm that the three active contacts, identified by three radiopaque markers, are parallel to the S1 to S4 lateral branch pathways. Care should be taken to ensure that the probe remains in contact with the sacral periosteum along its entire pathway. After the appropriate location is obtained, the Simplicity probe is connected to the RFA generator, and an appropriate heating sequence is chosen (Fig. 5.6). The RFA generator allows for procedure settings to be changed, including target temperature and lesion time. After this is done, typical RFA postoperative care should be undertaken, and follow-up should be scheduled.

STRIP LESIONING

Strip lesioning describes the process by which a bipolar strip lesion is created between two electrodes in the skin; the electrical current leapfrogs from one electrode to another, subsequently destroying the tissue adjacent to both probes.[10] For this procedure, two RFA probes within a distance of less than 5 to 6 mm of each other are placed, at which point a strip of heat is produced between them when electrical current is applied (Fig. 5.7). Like all RFA procedures, the patient is first positioned supine with a mobile C-arm in place for imaging. The area is prepped and draped in the usual sterile fashion. The grounding pad is applied as usual, away from any bony structures and locations where fluids may accumulate. An AP view is achieved, and radiopaque markers and skin markers are used to identify the top of the sacral ala lateral to the base of the S1 superior articular process of L5 to S1, as well as the caudal and lateral border of the S3 foramen. After the skin has been anesthetized, an RFA needle is advanced in conjunction with AP and lateral views until it contacts ostium on the dorsal surface of the sacrum. Confirmation that the RFA needle does not enter a foramen is paramount in the lateral view. A second RFA needle is then inserted in a similar fashion 5 to 10 mm caudal to the initial needle, creating the eventual boundaries (i.e., strips) of the first lesion. After the introducer is removed and local anesthetic (LA) is injected to numb the surrounding structures, ablation is initiated at 80°C to 85°C for 60 to

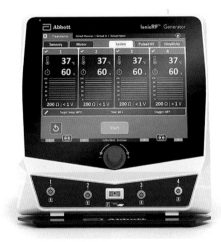

Fig. 5.6 Radiofrequency generator. (Reproduced with permission of Abbott, © 2022. All rights reserved.)

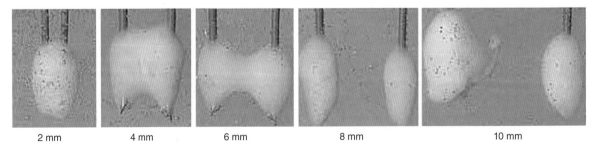

| 2 mm | 4 mm | 6 mm | 8 mm | 10 mm |

Fig. 5.7 Bipolar strip lesion created with two radiofrequency probes. (Source: Benzon HT, Rathmell JP, Wu CL, Turk DC, et al. *Practical Management of Pain.* 5th ed. St. Louis: Elsevier; 2014.)

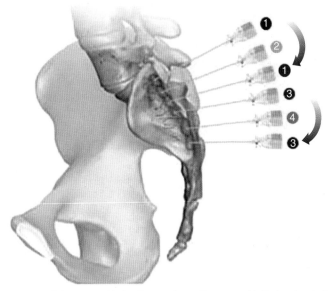

Fig. 5.8 Leapfrog technique using bipolar radiofrequency ablation (4 separate needles are used in the leapfrog technique). (Source: Used with permission by Abbott Laboratories.)

90 seconds. Next, the first needle is then removed and reinserted 5 to 10 mm caudal to the second needle toward the marker at the caudal and lateral border of the S3 foramen, and a second strip lesion is created as above (Fig. 5.8). This "leapfrog" technique continues to occur until there are five to seven continuous lesions that span the distance created by the two skin mark. This ensures that there has been ablation of the L5 dorsal ramus and the S1 to S3 lateral branches.[11] The probes are finally removed after ablation is complete, and typical RFA postprocedural care can take place.

RADIOFREQUENCY LESIONING

Radiofrequency lesioning is the most traditional and common way to perform RFA, and it uses either a thermal or water-cooled RFA probe. Water-cooled probes have the distinct advantage of a slower and more consistent heating pattern, thereby reducing the amount of scarring and necrosis that occurs, which can impede electrical current and can prevent a full ablation of the targeted nerve. To perform RFA lesioning, the patient is again positioned prone on an adjustable surgical table with a C-arm in place for imaging. The skin is prepped and draped in the usual sterile fashion.

With cooled RFA, the S1 to S3 sacral foramina are identified with AP oblique fluoroscopic images. A 25-gauge needle is then advanced cephalad and just lateral to each sacral foramen. This needle is used as guidance tool for the RFA introducer needles

(Fig. 5.9). Returning to the AP view, the skin is anesthetized with LA, the RFA introducer needles are advanced down to the sacral surface, and lateral views are taken to ensure correct depth of insertion. When the RFA probe (Figs. 5.10 and 5.11) is inserted, it should be suspended 2 to 3 mm above target nerve site. Ablation is then initiated at 60°C for 150 seconds. One can also use caudal sweeping of the introducer needle and RFA probe to create one or two additional lesions laterally along the S1 to S3 foramen.[12]

In contrast to cooled RFA, thermal RFA is typically only performed for ablation of the L4 to L5 and L5 to S1 dorsal rami. After the skin is anesthetized, an RFA needle is advanced until it is ideally 5 mm lateral to the sacral foramen between the 2 and 5 o'clock position on the right or the 7 and 10 o'clock position on the left. This will place the needle lateral to the connection between the sacral ala and the superior articular process of L5. A lateral view is acquired to ensure depth of insertion is correct and there is no insertion into the foramen. With the thermal radiofrequency probe specifically, the active lesioning site needs to overly the bone and ideally be parallel with the nerve trajectory to maximize ablation.

For all rami and lateral branches, there is first sensory stimulation before ablation, which is the main difference between radiofrequency lesioning and newer techniques such as Simplicity and strip lesioning. With the needle in place, the sensory stimulation setting is chosen, and a voltage (typically <0.6 V) is applied with the goal of reproducing SIJ pain. Then the voltage is increased to ensure there is absence of muscle contraction. Local anesthetic is injected, and lesions are created with either thermal (80°C for 90 seconds) or water-cooled (60°C for 150 seconds) probes. Like other techniques, the needles are removed, and typical postoperative care takes place.

Postoperative Considerations

Complications of SIJ RFA include damage to surrounding structures and nerves, including those essential to the structural integrity of the SIJ itself. There is also potential damage to other nerves necessary for

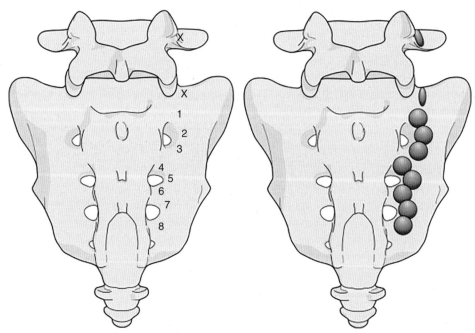

Fig. 5.9 Correct S1 to S4 lateral branch cooled radiofrequency probe placement (The numbers indicate the typical placement for probes in lateral branch RFA. The picture on the right shows the corresponding lesion created from each location).

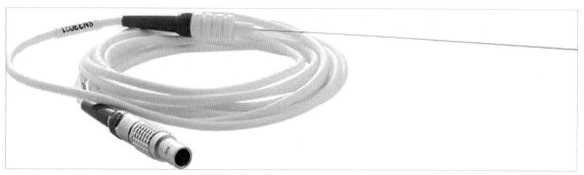

Fig. 5.10 Radiofrequency ablation probe.

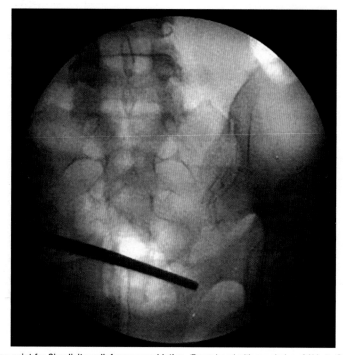

Fig. 5.11 Typical insertion point for Simplicity radiofrequency ablation.

motor function in the lower body because of the degree of anatomic variants that occur in the pelvic region. As with all surgeries, there is a risk of bleeding and infection, although these are exceedingly rare. The patient is instructed that the maximum effect of the ablation will not be felt for a number of weeks because the surrounding area is initially inflamed, and the nerve endings need to undergo Wallerian degeneration for full relief to occur.[13]

Management

Although RFA ablation remains a good choice for refractory SIJ pain, there are times when this will not provide complete relief for the patient even if they are a good candidate. At that point, management will include regular exercise, physical therapy, multimodal pain control, and potentially repeating RFA.

Conclusions

Chronic back pain is one of the most prevalent and debilitating diseases in the United States, and treatments commonly provide only temporary and incomplete relief of symptoms. The SIJ remains one of the main causes for chronic low back pain in the United States, and treatments are evolving quickly. Although it is relatively new, SIJ RFA provides a promising new technique for lesioning nerve roots responsible for back pain and is a promising option for many patients who have persistent back pain despite standard therapy regimens.

REFERENCES

1. Deyo RA, Tsui-Wu YJ. Descriptive epidemiology of low-back pain and its related medical care in the United States. *Spine (Phila Pa 1976)*. 1987;12(3):264-268.
2. Chuang C-W, Hung S-K, Pan P-T, Kao M-C. Diagnosis and interventional pain management options for sacroiliac joint pain. *Tzu Chui Medical J*. 2019;31(4):207-210.
3. Chou R, Loeser JD, Owens DK, et al. Interventional therapies, surgery, and interdisciplinary rehabilitation for low back pain. *Spine*. 2009;34:1066-1077.
4. Tuite MJ. Sacroiliac joint imaging. *Semin Musculoskelet Radiol*. 2008;12(1):72-82.
5. Hansen H, Manchikanti L, Simopoulos TT, et al. A systematic evaluation of the therapeutic effectiveness of sacroiliac joint interventions. *Pain Physician*. 2012;15:247-278.
6. Szadek KM, van der Wurff P, van Tulder MW, Zuurmond WW, Perez RS. Diagnostic validity of criteria for sacroiliac joint pain: a systematic review. *J Pain*. 2009;10:354-368.
7. Laslett M. Evidence-based diagnosis and treatment of the painful sacroiliac joint. *J Man Manip Ther*. 2008;16(3):142-152.
8. Maas ET, Ostelo RW, Niemisto L, et al. Radiofrequency denervation for chronic low back pain. *Cochrane Database Syst Rev*. 2015;2015(10):CD008572.
9. Yang AJ, Mccormick ZL, Zheng PZ, Schneider BJ. Radiofrequency ablation for posterior sacroiliac joint complex pain: a narrative review. *PM R*. 2019;11(suppl 1):S105-S113.
10. Hong K, Georgiades C. Radiofrequency ablation: mechanism of action and devices. *J Vasc Intervent Radiol*. 2010;21(suppl 8):S179-S186.
11. Cheng J, Chen SL, Zimmerman N, Dalton JE, LaSalle G, Rosenquist R. A new radiofrequency ablation procedure to treat sacroiliac joint pain. *Pain Physician*. 2016;19:603-615.
12. Ho K-Y, Hadi MA, Pasutharnchat K, Tan KH. Cooled radiofrequency denervation for treatment of sacroiliac joint pain: two-year results from 20 cases. *J Pain Res*. 2013;6:505-511.
13. Deer T, Leong MS, Buvanendran A, Gordin V, Kim P, Panchal S. *Comprehensive Treatment of Chronic Pain by Medical, Interventional, and Integrative Approaches: The American Academy of Pain Medicine Textbook on Patient Management*. New York: Springer; 2013.

Chapter 6

Peripheral Nerve Stimulation of the Sacroiliac Joint

Ryan Budwany, Alaa Abd-Elsayed, and Yeshvant Navalgund

Introduction

Peripheral nerve stimulation (PNS) is being explored for a variety of clinical indications, including plexus injuries, focal mononeuropathy, postamputation pain, back pain, sacroiliac joint pain (SIJ), headache, facial pain, and arm and limb pain.[1] PNS is an attractive treatment option for patients with SIJ pain who have failed more conservative treatments but who are not interested in a more invasive procedure because PNS is reversible, minimally invasive, and inherently less morbid than sacroiliac fusion.[1] This chapter focuses on treatment of patients with SIJ pain with PNS.

Pain and SIJ dysfunction is primarily caused by either a traumatic event through the disruption of normal anatomy or may develop over time through the degeneration of the structure listed below (Table 6.1).

Sacroiliac joint pain often presents with pain below the belt line with radiations into the groin and lower extremity, infrequently with radiations below the knee in the L5 to S1 dermatomal pattern (Figs. 6.1 and 6.2).

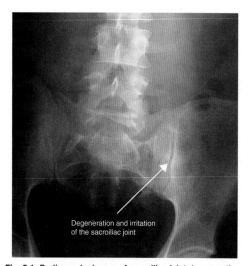

Fig. 6.1 Radiography image of sacroiliac joint degeneration.

Degeneration and irritation of the sacroiliac joint

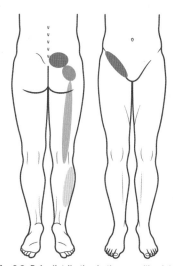

Fig. 6.2 Pain distribution in the sacroiliac joint.

TABLE 6.1 Frequent Causes of Sacroiliac Joint Pain	
Trauma or Joint Disruption	**Degeneration**
Car accident	Osteoarthritis
Fall on buttock	Infection
Crush injury	Previous lumbar spine surgery
Childbirth	Joint replacement surgery

Characteristics of SIJ pain[2] include
- Aching in quality
- Absence of burning quality
- Numbness and tingling
- Radiating down the posterior thigh to the posterior knee joint, glutes, sacrum, iliac crest, and sciatic distribution
- Worsening with static standing, bending forward, donning shoes or socks, crossing the leg, rising from a chair, or rolling in bed
- Relief with continuous change in position
- Typically, an absence of thigh pain, especially in older patients

Pain relief from PNS as sensed through paresthesia is mediated by A-beta fibers; however, the mechanism of segmental pain relief may share similar pathways with the spinal cord stimulation because the same A-beta fibers traverse the dorsal columns. It has been hypothesized that the PNS may affect local concentrations of biochemical mediators that enhance the pain response. Biochemical mediators of pain such as neurotransmitters and endorphins lead to increased local blood flow that may contribute to the development of chronic pain. Studies have suggested that the PNS may directly inhibit pain neurotransmission, possibly through alteration of local inflammatory mediators, as demonstrated by studies in healthy human volunteers, whereby elevated pain thresholds were observed during direct PNS. In peripheral nerve injury, ectopic discharges are transmitted by injured nerves, specifically low-threshold A-beta and high-threshold A-delta and C fibers, all of which may contribute to the generation of pain. It is postulated that PNS or direct nonpainful electrical stimulation may alter ectopic discharge, leading to decreased pain perception. Recent studies, however, have proposed that intact nerve fibers adjacent to the peripheral site of injury may be the culprits for pain generation via Wallerian degeneration.[3]

Indications

Peripheral nerve stimulation is indicated for pain management in adults who have severe intractable chronic pain of peripheral nerve origin, as the sole mitigating agent, or as an adjunct to other modes of therapy used in a multidisciplinary approach.[4]

Contraindications

Peripheral nerve stimulation is contraindicated in patients who are poor surgical candidates; pregnant; unable to understand or operate the system; will be exposed to shortwave, microwave, or ultrasound diathermy; have occupational exposure to high levels of nonionizing radiation; or have implanted cardiac systems.[4]

Perioperative Considerations

PATIENT SELECTION

Peripheral nerve stimulation is an appropriate treatment option for patients who maintain intractable pain even after conservative treatments such as SIJ injections or radiofrequency ablation of the SIJ.

Peripheral nerve stimulation can also be used earlier in the treatment paradigm when a patient does not want to have a more aggressive treatment such as fusion of the SIJ.

Preoperative Considerations

Table 6.2 describes some important aspects of the procedure setup.

TABLE 6.2	Procedure Setup
Anesthesia	Mild to moderate sedation. Deep sedation or general anesthesia should be avoided unless performed with nerve monitoring.
Positioning	Prone position with flattened or minimized lumbar lordosis No pressure on the belly or chest for ease of breathing for the patient
Antimicrobial Actions	Appropriate antibiotic is given before the start of the procedure. The target area is scrubbed with 2%–3% chlorhexidine/70% isopropyl alcohol solution. Three minutes is allowed for it to dry. Full surgical drapes are used, and the target skin area is covered with an antimicrobial incise drape (e.g., Ioban).

Procedure

Instructions for placement of PNS system are as follows:

1. Position patient in the prone position as shown in Figure 6.3.
2. Identify the path of middle cluneal nerve (MCN) as shown in Figure 6.4. The MCNs arise from the posterior rami of sacral spinal nerves (S1, S2, and S3). The site of MCN is caudal to the posterior superior iliac spine and at a slightly lateral point at the edge of the iliac crest.

3. Localize the track through the subcutaneous tissue (Fig. 6.5).
4. Insert a 14-gauge malleable needle to the endpoint as determined by the markings (Fig. 6.6). Block can also be performed under fluoroscopic guidance by blocking the nerves lateral to the sacral foramina as they exit (see Fig. 6.4)
5. Place leads as shown in Figure 6.7.
6. Withdraw needles past the lead contacts and test positioning for paresthesia over the painful area. Appropriately positioned quad and eight contact leads are shown in Figures 6.8 and 6.9.

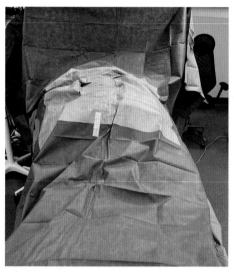

Fig. 6.3 A patient being prepared in the prone position.

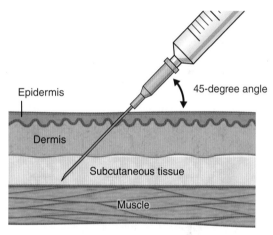

Fig. 6.5 Subcutaneous injection.

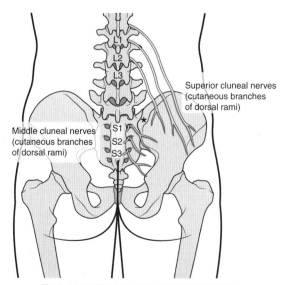

Fig. 6.4 Identification of the middle cluneal nerve.

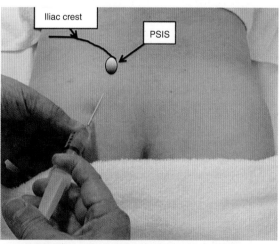

Fig. 6.6 Middle cluneal nerve blockage at the trigger point. *PSIS*, Posterior superior iliac spine. (Source: 2019 Springer Acta Neurochirurgica.)

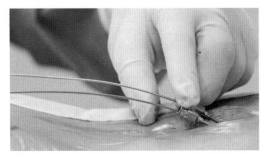

Fig. 6.7 Lead placement.

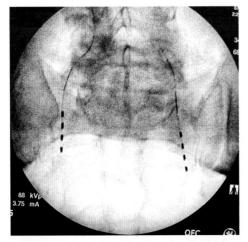

Fig. 6.8 Appropriately positioned quad contact leads.

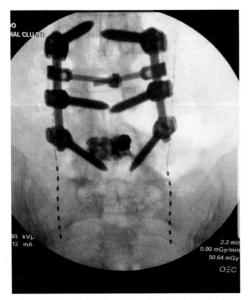

Fig. 6.9 Appropriately positioned eight contact leads.

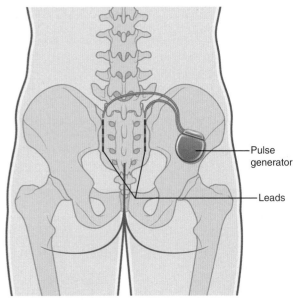

Fig. 6.10 Final placement of a peripheral nerve stimulation system.

7. If proceeding with a permanent implantation, incisions are made above and below the needles. Blunt dissection is performed around the needles. An incision is made to fit the pulse generator. A pocket is created with blunt dissection to fit the pulse generator. A strain relief loop is placed at each lead, and each lead is passed through a tunneling tool to the pulse generator pocket. The pulse generator is connected to the leads, and the incisions are closed (Fig. 6.10).

Postoperative Considerations

It is important as in all surgical procedures to consider postoperative care. After the needles are removed and the leads are secured to the patient, a protective bandage should be placed for the duration of the trial or during the healing after the implantation. Patients should be instructed to keep a cautious approach to activity, including a reduction in bending, twisting, and turning to prevent lead migration and promote capsular healing around the leads. This is usually for a period of 2 to 4 weeks.

TABLE 6.3 Postprocedure Care	
Acute recovery	Observation in recovery area until sedation wears off Brief neurologic examination is performed before discharge.
Discharge instructions	No need for postprocedure antibiotic coverage. Patient can ambulate freely once at home. Procedure pain should ease up in a few days.
Follow-up care	Patient should return in 2 weeks to evaluate the extent of symptom relief. At times, optimal functional improvement requires a course of physical therapy (PT) for muscle strengthening and conditioning. However, PT should not be considered until at least 8 weeks after the procedure to allow the devices to scar into place, thus minimizing the chance for dislodgement. A final assessment of patient improvement may not be feasible until a few months after the procedure.

Table 6.3 describes some important aspects of postprocedure care.

Management if Failed

Most instances of failure for this therapy are related to device malfunction, which may include lead fracture, lead displacement, or an electronic complication with the pulse generator. These issues can be resolved with replacement of the failed component.

Therapeutic failures should prompt the clinician to investigate other causes of the patient's symptoms. In rare circumstances, the stimulation system will require removal, and the patient should be referred for surgical intervention.

Postoperative infections can occur. Treatment necessitates removal of all device components and appropriate antibiotic treatment. In most instances, a new PNS system can be placed after the infection has cleared. Vigilance should be exercised to monitor patients closely postoperatively to ensure early detection of infection.

Clinical Pearls

- Ensure that the physical examination and symptoms correlate with a diagnosis of SIJ pain.
- Insert the introducer needle using fluoroscopy or ultrasonography to ensure an accurate trajectory.

- Be sure that during advancement of the needle in the subcutaneous tissue that the operator is able to palpate the needle at all times during advancement. This ensures security that the needle has not advanced to deeper tissue space.
- Verify with fluoroscopy that the needle is withdrawn past the lead electrodes to ensure proper contact with the MCN for stimulation.
- For a trial, use a securing anchor to the skin to ensure minimal lead migration.
- For a permanent implant, place an adequate strain relief loop to avoid lead migration.
- Typically, bulky anchors are not necessary because a good strain relief loop is sufficient.

REFERENCES

1. Guentchev M, Preuss C, Rink R, Peter L, Sailer MHM, Tuettenberg J. Long-term reduction of sacroiliac joint pain with peripheral nerve stimulation. *Oper Neurosurg (Hagerstown)*. 2017; 13(5):634-639.
2. Falowski S, Sayed D, Pope J, et al. A review and algorithm in the diagnosis and treatment of sacroiliac joint pain. *J Pain Res*. 2020;13:3337-3348.
3. Chakravarthy K, Nava A, Christo PJ, Williams K. Review of recent advances in peripheral nerve stimulation (PNS). *Curr Pain Headache Rep*. 2016;20(11):60.
4. Stimwave Technologies. *StimQ PNS System Implantation of Trial Lead. Instructions for Use*. Available at: https://thepaincenterinc.com/Portals/0/PDFs/StimQ-PNS.pdf.

Chapter 7

Sacroiliac Joint Posterior Fusion

Alaa Abd-Elsayed and Ahish Chitneni

Introduction

The sacroiliac joint (SIJ) functions in transferring the load between the spine and the lower extremities and acts as a shock absorber for the spine. The structure is bordered by sacroiliac ligaments on both the anterior and posterior aspects. Many studies have associated the dysfunction of the SIJ as a source of back pain with the prevalence ranging from 10% to 38% of cases of low back pain.[1] Conservative measures of treatment that can be considered include medications, activity modification, physical therapy, use of intraarticular steroid injections for pain relief, and radiofrequency ablation. In cases in which pain continues to persist despite conservative measures, surgical stabilization or SIJ fusion can be considered. Previously, SIJ fusion was conducted under open surgery with hardware placement. Various studies have shown that patients who underwent this procedure continued to have persistent severe pain at follow-up.[2] Additionally, in an open fusion procedure, various pitfalls exist such as the length of the procedure, associated blood loss, length of hospitalization postoperatively, and increased levels of complications.[3] In recent years, the development of a posterior approach to SIJ fusion with the use of cortical allograft placement and a drill-less method allows for a safer and more effective approach to SIJ fusion.

Anatomic Considerations

In essence, the SIJs (SIJ) articulate both the sacrum and the ilium. SIJs are essential joints that aid in transferring the load between the spine and the lower extremities.[4] Functionally, the SIJ acts as a shock absorber for the spine. The SIJ consists of a synovial joint and a syndesmosis, which are the intra- and extraarticular parts, respectively.[5] The SIJ has a surrounding fibrous capsule with synovial fluid between the surfaces.[6] Various ligaments exist around the SIJ, which at times may be sources of pain and inflammation. The sacroiliac ligament connects the sacrum to the ilium, and the posterior sacroiliac ligament connects the posterior superior iliac spine to the iliac crest to segments of the sacrum.[6] Additional ligaments include the sacrotuberous ligament and the sacrospinous ligament. The sacrotuberous ligaments connect to the aforementioned posterior sacroiliac ligament, and the sacrospinous ligament originates in the ischial spine and attaches to the lateral aspect of the sacrum.[6]

Various sources of blood supply to the SIJ exist. As for the blood supply, the internal iliac artery innervates the anterior aspect of the SIJ, and the superior gluteal artery can innervate the posterior aspect of the SIJ.[6] Additionally, the median sacral artery and lateral sacral artery originate from the internal iliac artery and supply the SIJ.

As for the nerve innervation to the SIJ, research has shown that there is variability among different patients in the innervation of the SIJ.[7] Despite the variability, in general, the innervation of the SIJ and surrounding ligaments is innervated anteriorly from the branches of the ventral rami of L4 and L5, branches of gluteal nerves, and the obturator nerve. In the posterior aspect, the innervation consists of the dorsal rami of S1 to S3 and the L5 dorsal ramus.[8]

Patient Selection and Indications

Various selection indicators and indications exist for a patient to qualify for a posterior SIJ fusion. In general, for a patient to qualify for a posterior SIJ fusion, the patient must have history and physical examination findings of sacroiliitis, must have failed conservative management, and must have undergone a diagnostic local anesthetic SIJ injection. In general, the physical examination consists of various maneuvers (e.g., SIJ distraction test, the thigh thrust, the Gaenslen's maneuver, the compression test, the FABER [flexion, abduction, and external rotation] test) to diagnose sacroiliitis, and diagnosis typically requires positive findings in three of five provocative maneuvers.[9] Additionally, patients typically undergo a diagnostic SIJ injection to confirm that the source of pain is the SIJ. In this procedure, the patient undergoes the injection of local anesthetic via fluoroscopic guidance at the site of the SIJ to assess for greater than 50% pain relief.[9] Additionally, patients with SIJ dysfunction typically have symptoms consisting of dull low back pain, sciatica-type symptoms, worsening pain with activity, an increased amount of pain in the morning, and muscle tightness in the bilateral hips or buttocks.

Contraindications

Various contraindications exist that may exclude a patient from undergoing an SIJ posterior fusion. Most important, patients who have not attempted conservative management with medications and physical therapy typically do not qualify for the procedure. Additionally, patients who may have insufficient pain relief from the diagnostic fluoroscopic-guided injection of local anesthetic to the SIJ do not qualify for SIJ fusion. Other contraindications to undergoing the procedure include any signs of systematic or spine infections, spinal malignancies, metastatic malignancy, pregnancy, and increased risk of bleeding caused by bleeding disorders.

Description of the Procedure

Various procedure methods have been described to conduct a posterior SIJ fusion. In the procedure, the patient typically lies down prone under a fluoroscopy machine. Before the start of the procedure, all the instruments shown in Figure 7.1 should be confirmed, including the Steinmann guide pin, implant inserter, joint decorticator, outside dilator, and inside dilator. A 22-gauge needle is used to administer local lidocaine before starting the procedure. After successful local anesthetic administration, a 2- to 3-cm stab incision is made along the skin. After the incision is made, the

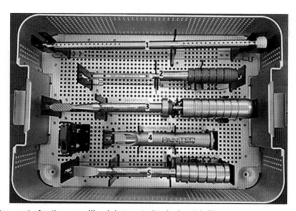

Instruments

1. Guide pin storage tube
2. Implant inserter
3. Joint decorticator
4. Outside dilator and
   working channel
5. Inside dilator

Fig. 7.1 Instruments for the sacroiliac joint posterior fusion (LinQ).

Steinmann pin is advanced into the anterior cortical line of the SIJ as seen in Figures 7.2 and 7.3 in the lateral and anteroposterior views, respectively, and schematically in Figure 7.4. After proper placement of the pin under fluoroscopic guidance, the inside dilator is slid into the outside dilator, and the dilators are advanced down the Steinmann pin until localized to the SIJ as seen in Figures 7.5 and 7.6. After proper advancement, the internal dilator is removed, and a decorticator (see Fig. 7.1) is placed at the site of the outside dilator and advanced with the use of a mallet as seen in Figures 7.7 and 7.8. After proper placement

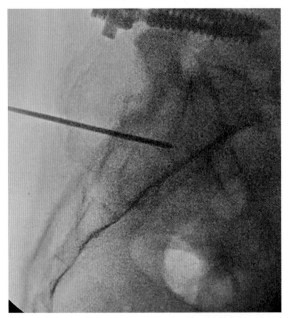

Fig. 7.2 Lateral view of Steinmann pin placement.

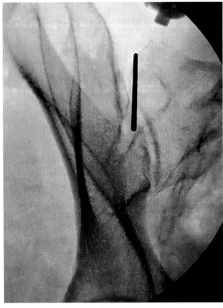

Fig. 7.3 Anteroposterior view of Steinmann pin placement.

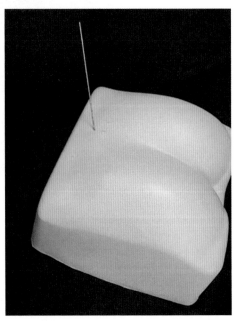

Fig. 7.4 View of the Steinmann pin placement.

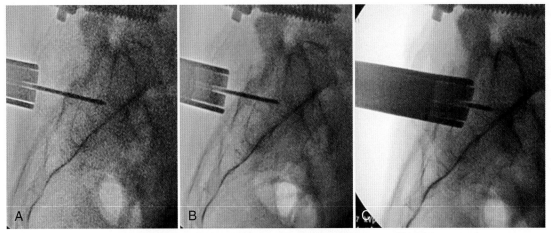

Fig. 7.5 A–C, Lateral views of the internal dilator seated in the sacroiliac joint.

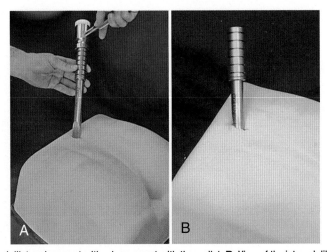

Fig. 7.6 A, View of the internal dilator placement with advancement with the mallet. **B,** View of the internal dilator in place after positioning.

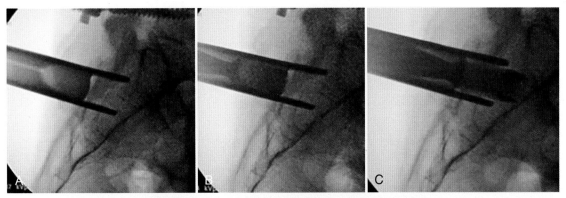

Fig. 7.7 A–C, Lateral views of decorticator placement and advancement.

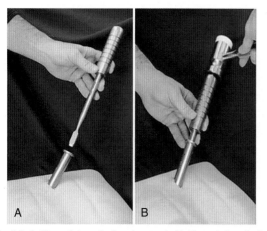

Fig. 7.8 A, View of decorticator placement. **B,** View of decorticator placement and advancement with the use of a mallet.

of the decorticator is confirmed under fluoroscopy, the decorticator is removed with the use of the mallet, and the allograft device is placed into the SIJ as seen in Figures 7.9 and 7.10. After confirmation of the placement, all the devices are removed, and a final confirmation is done under fluoroscopy to confirm the placement of the allograft as seen in the lateral and anteroposterior views in Figure 7.11. After confirmation, irrigation of the incision is conducted, and 2-0 Vicryl sutures are used for the closure of the open wound with dressing applied at the incision site.

Another similar procedure consists of the use of two cortical allografts placed orthogonally to prevent potential migration of the allografts.[10] In this procedure, compared with the placement of one Steinmann

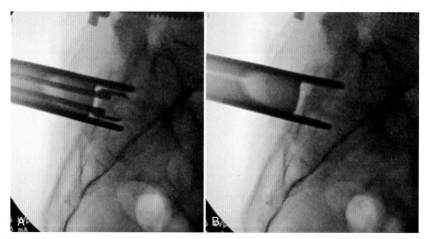

Fig. 7.9 A, Lateral view of the placement of the allograft prior to completion. **B,** Lateral view of the placement of the allograft.

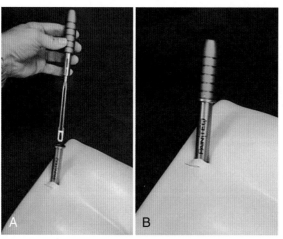

Fig. 7.10 A, View of the placement of the allograft implantation before advancement. **B,** View of the placement of the allograft implantation after advancement.

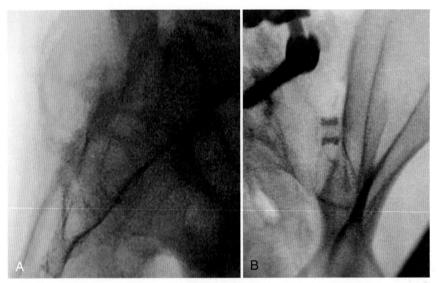

Fig. 7.11 Lateral (**A**) and anteroposterior (**B**) views of the final confirmation of allograft placement.

in the procedure described earlier, two pins are placed as seen in Figures 7.12 and 7.13. After confirmation of proper placement of the pins under fluoroscopy, the inside dilator is slid into the outside dilator and advanced down to the location of the SIJ

as seen in Figure 7.14. Similar to the procedure described previously, the allograft is placed at the site of SIJ as seen in Figure 7.15, and a final confirmation of allograft placement is conducted as seen in Figure 7.16

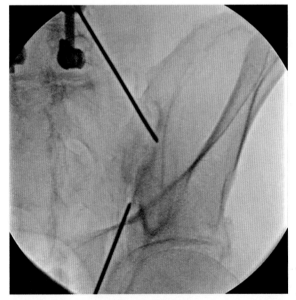

Fig. 7.12 Anteroposterior view of two Steinmann pin placement in the sacroiliac joint.

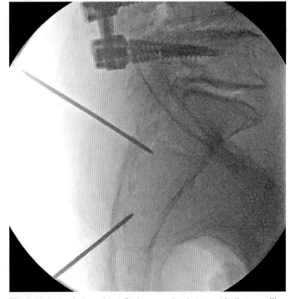

Fig. 7.13 Lateral view of two Steinmann pin placement in the sacroiliac joint.

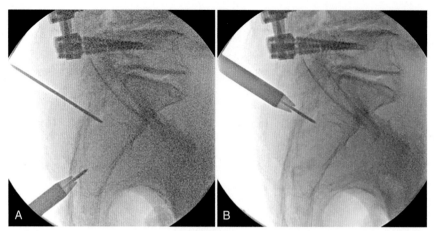

Fig. 7.14 A, Lateral view of internal dilator placement at the site of Steinmann pin #1. **B,** Lateral view of internal dilator placement at the site of Steinmann pin #2.

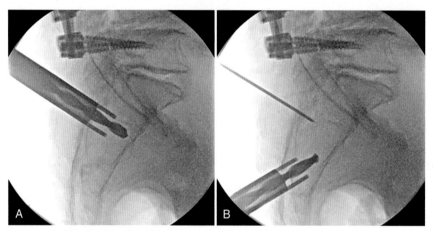

Fig. 7.15 A, Allograft placement at the site of location #1 in the sacroiliac joint. **B,** Allograft placement at the site of location #2 in the sacroiliac joint.

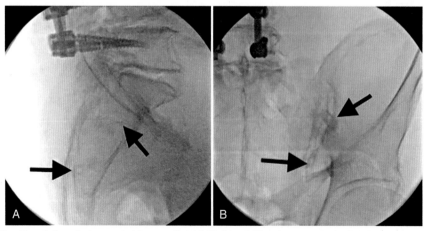

Fig. 7.16 Final confirmation of allograft placement at the sacroiliac joint in lateral (**A**) and anteroposterior (**B**) views. *Arrows* indicate the location of sacroiliac joint allograft placement.

Intraoperative Complications

As with any interventional procedure, various intraoperative complications may exist. In general, some complications include the risk of bleeding, muscle damage, nerve damage, and worsening of SIJ pain. In many of the studies conducted, adverse effects during the procedure were noted to be extremely rare. One large-scale multicenter retrospective analysis assessed 110 patients who had received SIJ posterior fusion. In the review, none of the patients required intraoperative blood transfusion or products or an extended length of hospital stay, and no evidence of localized infection, systemic infection, or neurologic injury was reported.[9] In one case described in the review, a patient had a significant device migration, which presented as worsening of SIJ pain and required repositioning of the allograft device.[9]

Postoperative Care

Typical postoperative care for SIJ posterior fusion procedure includes the application of an adhesive bandage at the puncture site. In general, after the completion of the fluoroscopic-guided procedure, the patient is transferred to a recovery room for monitoring of vital signs, for monitoring of any allergic reaction to the products used, and for observing any signs of decompensation. Additionally, typically postoperatively, patients are recommended to avoid driving or operating machinery for 24 hours, avoiding any rigorous physical activity for 24 hours. The adhesive bandage at the puncture site is removed after 24 hours. Additionally, any postoperative pain at the puncture site can be managed with the use of an ice pack and the use of nonsteroidal antiinflammatory drugs and other over-the-counter medications. Overall, in general, patients are typically discharged on the same day of the procedure with scheduled postprocedure follow-up appointments.

General Considerations

Various studies have been conducted on the use of SIJ fusion for the treatment of patients with SIJ dysfunction. One of the studies conducted was a study by Sayed et al.,[9] which was a multicenter retrospective analysis of the long-term efficacy and safety of the SIJ fusion device. In the study, a retrospective study 12 months after the LinQ procedure was conducted. Of the 110 patients assessed who received the SIJ fusion, 50 patients were evaluated because of sufficient data with outcomes over 12 months after the procedure. Results showed that the average pain numerical rating scale (NRS) score was 6.98 before the SIJ fusion with the average score at 3.06 at the follow-up visit. Additionally, all 50 patients were assessed, and all the procedures were completed with no complications or adverse events. In one case, one of the patients had an allograft migration, which required a repeat procedure for allograft fixture.

Another study conducted by Deer et al.[11] was a multicenter retrospective observational study on the use of the posterior SIJ fusion, and it assessed pain relief in patients. In the study, a total of 111 patients who underwent a posterior SIJ fusion were assessed. Results showed that the mean reported pain relief was 67.6% over the course of 291 days.

Additional studies that discuss the use of posterior SIJ fusion include retrospective studies conducted by Patterson et al.[12] and Mann et al.[13] Both these studies discussed the use of the ConcerLoc procedure, and the Patterson et al.[12] study assessed 21 patients who underwent the procedure. In this study, there was an overall reduction of pain at 73.2% at the 12-week follow-up appointment and an average 6.29 reduction in the NRS score. In the Mann et al.[13] study, 10 patients were assessed who underwent the CornerLoc posterior SIJ fusion procedure. In this study, at the 12-week follow-up appointment, the average NRS score reduction was at 4.6, and an overall decrease in 62.3% pain relief was found in the patients assessed.

Overall, all of these studies lack a true control group and are all retrospective studies conducted on patients who underwent various types of posterior SIJ fusion procedures. In the future, further large-scale randomized studies on the use of the procedures with a control group need to be conducted. In addition, many of these studies used different procedures and techniques, and further studies comparing the two procedures and the assessment of complications, efficacy, and pain relief need to be conducted.

REFERENCES

1. Yoshihara H. Sacroiliac joint pain after lumbar/lumbosacral fusion: current knowledge. *Eur Spine J.* 2012;21(9):1788-1796.
2. Schütz U, Grob D. Poor outcome following bilateral sacroiliac joint fusion for degenerative sacroiliac joint syndrome. *Acta Orthop Belg.* 2006;72(3):296-308.
3. Ou-Yang DC, York PJ, Kleck CJ, Patel VV. Diagnosis and management of sacroiliac joint dysfunction. *J Bone Joint Surg Am.* 2017;99(23):2027-2036.
4. Vleeming A, Schuenke MD, Masi AT, Carreiro JE, Danneels L, Willard FH. The sacroiliac joint: an overview of its anatomy, function and potential clinical implications. *J Anat.* 2012;221(6):537-567.
5. Roberts SL. Sacroiliac joint anatomy. *Phys Med Rehabil Clin N Am.* 2021;32(4):703-724.
6. Wong M, Sinkler MA, Kiel J. Anatomy, abdomen and pelvis, sacroiliac joint. [Updated 2021 Aug 11]. In: *StatPearls* [Internet]. Treasure Island, FL: StatPearls Publishing; 2022.
7. Roberts SL, Burnham RS, Ravichandiran K, Agur AM, Loh EY. Cadaveric study of sacroiliac joint innervation: implications for diagnostic blocks and radiofrequency ablation. *Reg Anesth Pain Med.* 2014;39(6):456-464.
8. Ikeda R. Innervation of the sacroiliac joint. Macroscopical and histological studies. *Nihon Ika Daigaku Zasshi.* 1991;58(5):587-596.
9. Sayed D, Balter K, Pyles S, Lam CM. A multicenter retrospective analysis of the long-term efficacy and safety of a novel posterior sacroiliac fusion device. *J Pain Res.* 2021;14:3251-3258.
10. CornerLoc. *For Physicians.* Available at: https://cornerloc.com/for-si-joint-physicians.
11. Deer TR, Rupp A, Budwany R, et al. Pain relief salvage with a novel minimally invasive posterior sacroiliac joint fusion device in patients with previously implanted pain devices and therapies. *J Pain Res.* 2021;14:2709-2715.
12. Patterson D, Wilits M, Fiks V, et al. Pain reduction and functional improvement after posterior approach SI stabilization and fusion with specialized graft: a case series. Paper presented at the CASIPP Annual Meeting; 2018.
13. Mann D, Willits M, Fiks V, et al. Pain reduction at 12 months after posterior approach SI stabilization and fusion with specialized graft: 10 case series. Paper presented at the ASPN Annual Meeting; 2019.

Chapter 8

Lateral Sacroiliac Joint Fusion

Hamid R. Abbasi, Alaa Abd-Elsayed, and Nicholas R. Storlie

Introduction

Sacroiliac joint (SIJ) disease has been increasingly recognized as a common contributor to many cases of lower back pain (LBP) and radiculopathy, with a prevalence estimated at between 13% and 30% in patients with LBP.[1,2] Although the cause of SIJ pain is not fully understood, it is thought to be inflammation and injury to nociceptors throughout the joint capsule and ligaments following trauma or repeated stresses.[3] SIJ fusion alleviates pain through providing stability to the joint and preventing excessive motion. Surgical treatment of SIJ pathologies through fusion of the ilium and sacrum has been demonstrated to significantly decrease pain and disability with appropriately selected patients using several techniques.[4,5] Although historically performed through both open and minimally invasive techniques, less invasive methods of fusion have become the dominant method of SIJ fusion.[6]

This chapter discusses minimally invasive lateral approaches to SIJ fusion tat attempt to fuse the bone by placement of an implant through the ilium and across the SIJ. These surgeries have short operative times, are associated with low blood loss, and can be performed in an outpatient setting.[7] Common methods of achieving fusion through a lateral approach include percutaneous placement of bone plugs or screws with bone graft; the latter is discussed in this chapter.

Indications

Sacroiliac joint fusion is indicated for the treatment of SIJ pain for patients with low back and/or buttock pain who meet *all* of the following criteria:

1. Underwent and failed a minimum of 6 months of intensive nonoperative treatment that includes medication optimization, activity modification, and active physical therapy
2. Report unilateral and/or bilateral pain that is at or near the L5 vertebrae, localized over the posterior SIJ, and consistent with SIJ pain. (Pain radiating down the leg does not rule out SIJ disease.)
3. Report localized tenderness with palpation of the posterior SIJ and/or groin in the absence of tenderness of similar severity elsewhere and other obvious sources for the pain do not exist (Fortin's test).
4. Have a positive response to the thigh thrust test *or* compression test *and* two of the following additional provocation tests:
   a. Gaenslen's test
   b. Distraction test
   c. Patrick's sign
   d. FABER (flexion, abduction, and external rotation) test
   e. Fortin's test
5. Have an absence of generalized pain behavior (e.g., somatoform disorder) and generalized pain disorders (e.g., fibromyalgia). If these are present, diagnoses have been ruled out as the source of the patient's pain.
6. Diagnostic imaging studies that include all of the following:
   a. Imaging of the SIJ that excludes the presence of destructive lesions or inflammatory arthropathy that would not be properly addressed by percutaneous SIJ fusion
   b. Imaging of the ipsilateral hip to rule out osteoarthritis
   c. Imaging of the lumbar spine to rule out neural compression and other degenerative conditions that can cause low back or buttock pain

7. Have at least 75% reduction of pain for the expected duration of the anesthetic (hours to days) used following an image-guided, contrast-enhanced SI injection on two or three separate occasions

Contraindications

Sacroiliac joint fusion for SIJ pain is NOT indicated in any of the following scenarios, except in specific circumstances when other pathologies have been investigated separately and ruled out as a source of pain:

1. Any case that does not fulfill *all* of the above criteria
2. The presence of systemic arthropathy such as ankylosing spondylitis or rheumatoid arthritis
3. The presence of generalized pain behavior or generalized pain disorder
4. The presence of infection, tumor, or fracture
5. The presence of neural compression as seen on magnetic resonance imaging or computed tomography that correlates with the patient's symptoms and is most likely the source of their pain

Preoperative Considerations

Routine patient evaluation for risk of infection, use of anticoagulation, and addressing all comorbidities that may impact the operative course should be done.

Preoperatively, the patient is induced and placed in the prone position on a Jackson table. The area around the patient's SIJ is prepared, and the draping is performed before surgery. Intraoperatively, 1% lidocaine with epinephrine and 0.25% Marcaine plain mixed 1:1 is injected at the skin where the incision will be made.

Postoperative Care

The patient is usually discharged within 4 hours of the case, almost always the same day as the surgery. The patient is discharged with pain medication and muscle relaxants. If there is excess bleeding, an ACE wrap is used to compress the surgical site. Patients are typically able to walk with a walker immediately after surgery with toe-touch weight-bearing restrictions for 2 to 4 weeks.

Complications

Complications of minimally invasive SIJ fusion include the following:

1. Rare cases of higher blood loss if the iliac crest is violated during the procedure. This is treated with an ACE bandage wrap around the patient's torso and the surgical site.
2. Loosening of screws requiring revision, mostly seen in cases of falls after the procedure before fusion has been achieved. Serial diagnostic SIJ injections are performed before revision to confirm that hardware loosening is responsible for clinical symptoms.
3. In our practice, we observed one case of gluteal hematoma requiring evacuation that was later found to have an iliac artery pseudoaneurysm requiring coiling.[7]
4. Wound dehiscence has been rarely observed and treated by secondary intention with local wound care.

Background

IMAGING AND ANATOMY

Three radiography positions are used in this technique: lateral (Fig. 8.1), inlet (Fig. 8.2), and outlet (Fig. 8.3). The inlet view displays the true axial view of the first three sacral vertebrae and is achieved by tilting the x-ray tube cephalad (Fig. 8.4). The outlet view is the true anterior view of the sacrum and is achieved by tilting the x-ray beam caudally (Fig. 8.5).

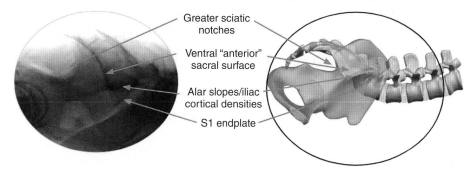

Greater sciatic notches

Ventral "anterior" sacral surface

Alar slopes/iliac cortical densities

S1 endplate

Fig. 8.1 Lateral view of sacroiliac joint anatomy on radiography *(left)* and on a model *(right)*.

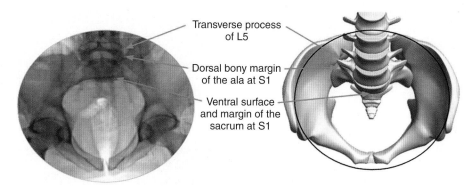

Transverse process of L5

Dorsal bony margin of the ala at S1

Ventral surface and margin of the sacrum at S1

Fig. 8.2 Inlet view of sacroiliac joint anatomy on radiography *(left)* and on a model *(right)*.

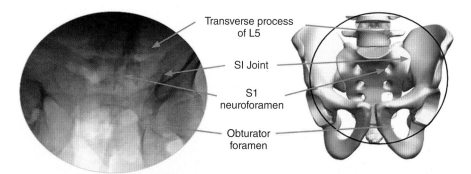

Transverse process of L5

SI Joint

S1 neuroforamen

Obturator foramen

Fig. 8.3 Outlet view of sacroiliac joint on radiography *(left)* and on a model *(right)*.

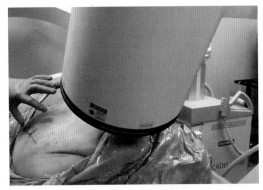

Fig. 8.4 Positioning of the C-arm for the inlet view.

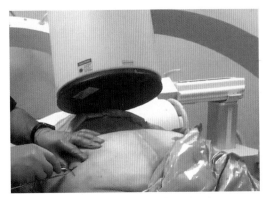

Fig. 8.5 Positioning of C-arm for outlet view.

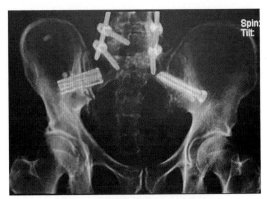

Fig. 8.6 Three-dimensional visualization of a patient with the sacroiliac joint fused bilaterally with distinct systems both using a lateral transiliac approach. On the *left*, L&K Biomed PathLoc-SI screws are shown. On the *right*, Zyga SImmetry screws are shown.

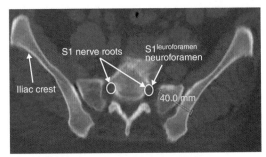

Fig. 8.7 Axial computed tomography slice showing the first sacral foramen.

Transiliac Arch Screws

Postoperative imaging demonstrating completed SIJ fusion using this technique is seen in Figure 8.6.

PREOPERATIVE PLANNING

The appropriate size of implant should be selected before surgery. The implant size can be estimated by measuring the length of a line perpendicular to the outer boundary of the ilium to the first sacral foramen in the axial view (Fig. 8.7).

TARGETING

The patient is placed in the prone position on the operative table. C-arm fluoroscopy is used to provide imaging during the procedure. Neuromonitoring may be used to monitor muscles throughout the procedure for increased safety.

Lateral fluoroscopy should be used to visualize the trochanteric notch and ala (Fig. 8.8).

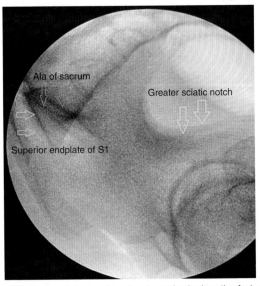

Fig. 8.8 The true lateral pelvic view is attained when the features noted are aligned.

Mark the sacral shadow on the skin and draw a line from the sacral promontory to the middle of the sciatic notch using a guide pin and marking pen. The skin incision is made 1 inch perpendicularly above this line at the middle of the sciatic notch (Figs. 8.9 and 8.10).

Insert the blunt end of the guide pin lateral to medial through the incision and place guide pin on the ilium about 1 inch caudal to the shadow of the ala and aligned with the anterior wall of the sacrum for the first screw placed (Fig. 8.11). We make contact with

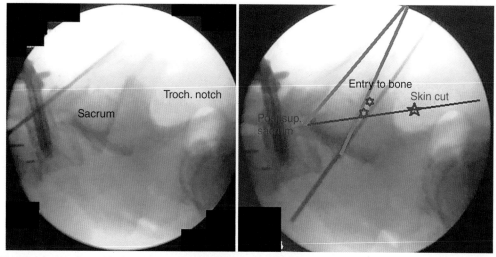

Fig. 8.9 Lateral radiographic view demonstrating how to determine the incision point and desired entry points into the ilium.

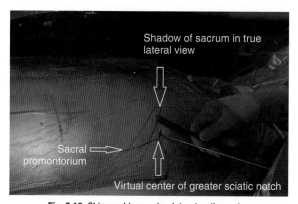

Fig. 8.10 Skin markings using lateral radiography.

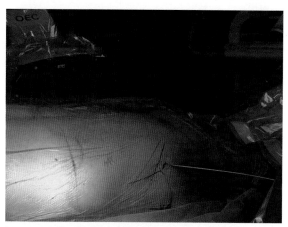

Fig. 8.11 Guide pin inserted at the virtual center of the greater sciatic notch.

the iliac crest so that it aligns with the S1 to S2 foramen in the lateral view (Fig. 8.12).

Use the lateral view to visualize placement of the guide pin. After docking the blunt end of the guide pin, place the first dilator (Ø7.95 mm) over the guide pin and dock on the lateral edge of the ilium to stabilize the approach trajectory and switch to the sharp end of the guide pin (Fig. 8.13). When the entry point is established just cranial to the S1 to S2 foramen, the pelvic inlet (Fig. 8.14) and outlet (Fig. 8.15) views are used to adjust the guidewire trajectory.

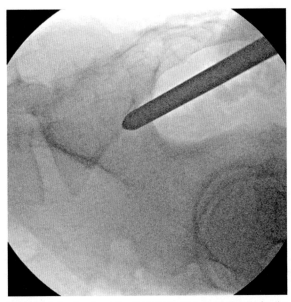

Fig. 8.14 Lateral radiography showing desired docking point for the first dilator.

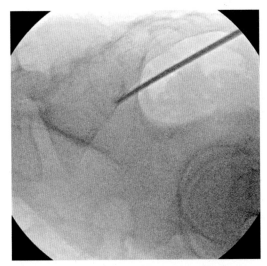

Fig. 8.12 Lateral image of the docked guide pin.

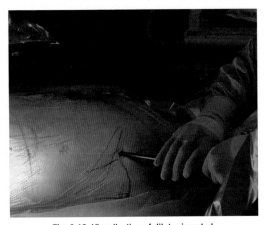

Fig. 8.13 Visualization of dilator inserted.

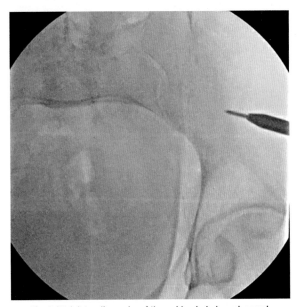

Fig. 8.15 Inlet radiography of the guide pin being advanced.

Remove the guide pin when the dilator is set in the correct and stable position. Reinsert the guide pin with the trocar end entering first and advance to the lateral edge of the ilium. The guide pin is used for initial targeting to reduce the risk of vascular injury to branches of gluteal arteries (Fig. 8.16).

Using a pin driver, advance the guide pin across the ilium across the SIJ and into the sacrum while in the inlet view (Figs. 8.17 to 8.19).

Insert a second dilator over the first down to the iliac crest (Figs. 8.20 and 8.21). Insert the insertion guide over the second dilator (Figs. 8.22 and 8.23). Use a mallet to dock the insertion guide against the ilium and remove both inner dilators (Fig. 8.24).

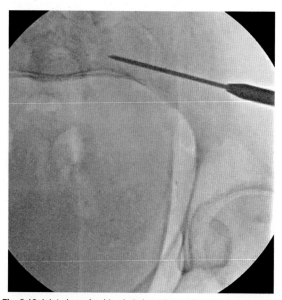

Fig. 8.18 Inlet view of guide pin being advanced across the sacroiliac joint using a drill.

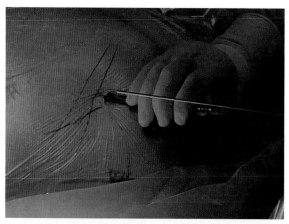

Fig. 8.16 The guide pin is flipped and inserted thread end first.

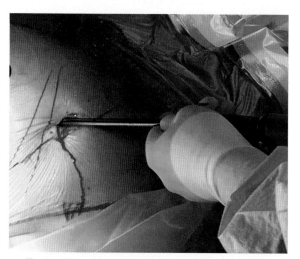

Fig. 8.17 The guide pin being drilled past the sacroiliac joint.

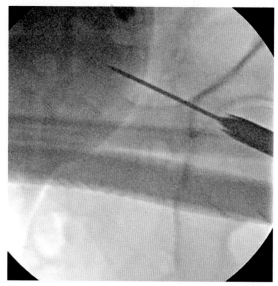

Fig. 8.19 Outlet view of the dilator advanced through the sacroiliac joint.

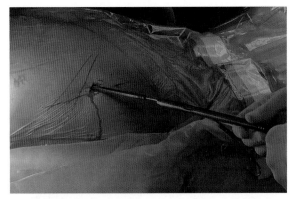

Fig. 8.20 The second dilator being inserted over the first.

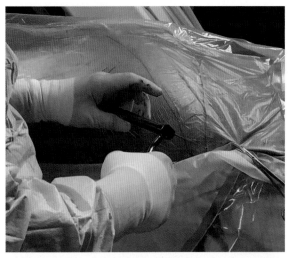

Fig. 8.22 The insertion guide being inserted over the second dilator.

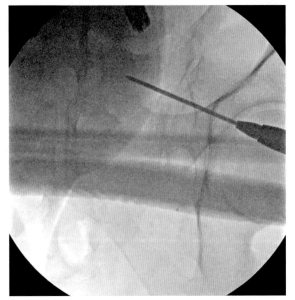

Fig. 8.21 Outlet view of the second dilator advanced through the sacroiliac joint.

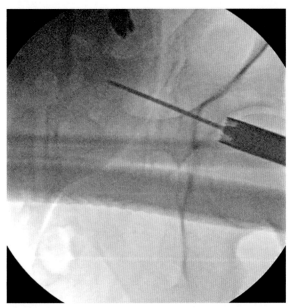

Fig. 8.23 Outlet view of the insertion guide advanced through the sacroiliac joint.

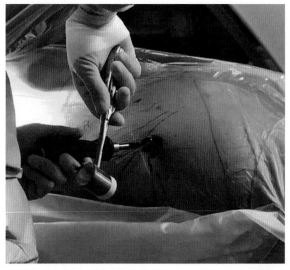

Fig. 8.24 A mallet is used to dock the insertion guide against the ilium.

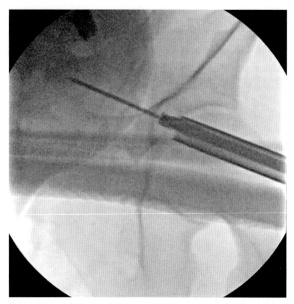

Fig. 8.26 A Ø7.8-mm drill is inserted through the sacroiliac joint.

Use drills and taps as needed to prepare for the insertion of the screw. In this case, a Ø7.8-mm and then a Ø10.3-mm drill are inserted through the SIJ to prepare for the Ø12-mm screw (Figs. 8.25 to 8.28).

After you have prepared an entrance, the arch screw can be inserted until the screw is centered between the sacrum and the ilium (Figs. 8.29 to 8.31). The correct placement of the screw is determined by

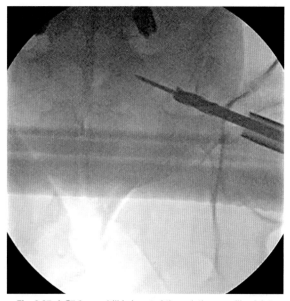

Fig. 8.27 A Ø7.8-mm drill is inserted through the sacroiliac joint.

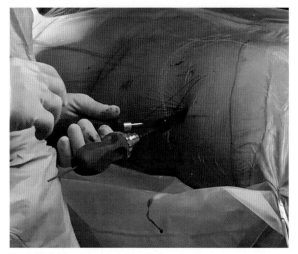

Fig. 8.25 Drills are inserted through the sacroiliac joint to prepare for the 12-mm screw.

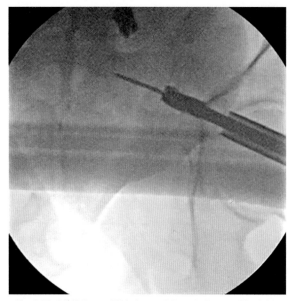

Fig. 8.28 A Ø10.3-mm drill is inserted through the sacroiliac joint.

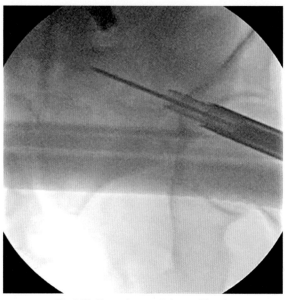

Fig. 8.30 The arch screw being positioned.

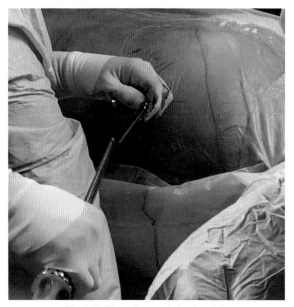

Fig. 8.29 The arch screw being inserted.

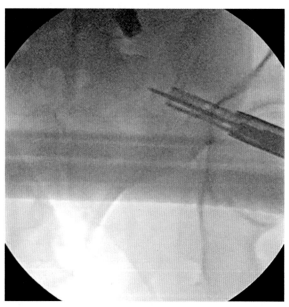

Fig. 8.31 The arch screw is centered between the sacrum and ilium.

feeling when the screw has entered the cortical bone on the posterior wall of the sacrum. The surgeon will feel resistance on passing through the iliac cortical bone of the SIJ and subsequently when the screw passes into the cortical bone of the sacrum. There will be less resistance as the screw passes through the sacral vertebral bodies until the screw approaches the cortical bone of the posterior sacral wall. When this resistance is felt, the screw is given another half turn, which completes screw placement (Fig. 8.32).

After the screw is placed, the bone graft is inserted into the center of the hollow screw (Figs. 8.33 and 8.34).

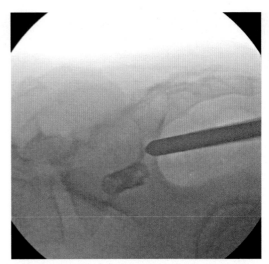

Fig. 8.34 Lateral view of the first arch screw placement.

SECOND SCREW PLACEMENT

The second screw placement is similar to the placement of the first screw, but the guide pin is docked 1 to 1.5 cm caudally along the line of the sacrum (Figs. 8.35 to 8.45).

Trident Sacroiliac Joint Screw System

The Trident SIJ screw system is a relatively new SIJ fusion system using a lateral approach similar to that

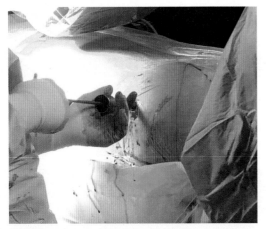

Fig. 8.32 The arch screw is given one last half turn after the correct positioning has been determined.

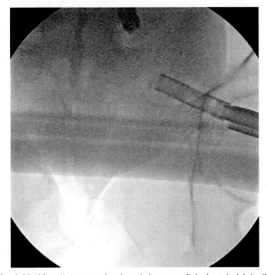

Fig. 8.33 After the screw is placed, bone graft is inserted into the center of the hollow screw.

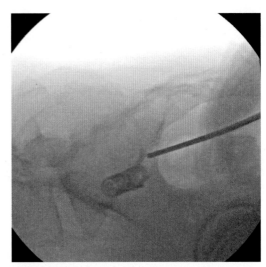

Fig. 8.35 The guide pin is docked 1 to 1.5 cm caudally along the line of the sacrum.

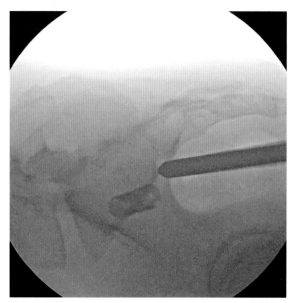

Fig. 8.36 Docking of the dilator and guide pin in the lateral view.

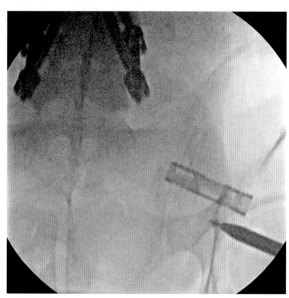

Fig. 8.38 Docking of the dilator and guidewire in the outlet view.

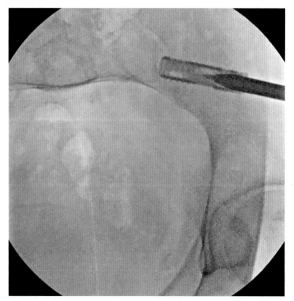

Fig. 8.37 Docking of the guide pin and dilator in the inlet view.

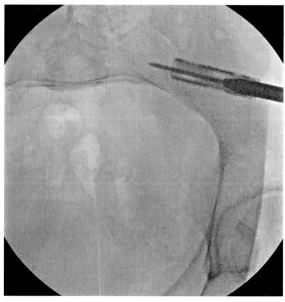

Fig. 8.39 The guide pin advances through the sacroiliac joint in the inlet view.

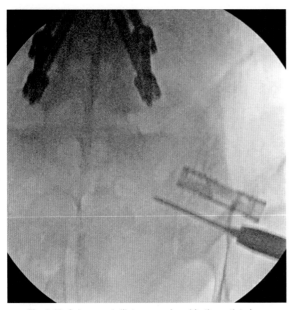

Fig. 8.40 Subsequent dilators are placed in the outlet view.

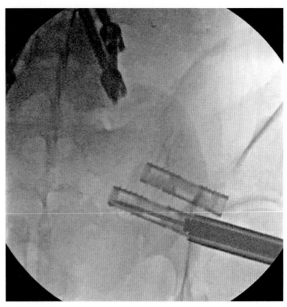

Fig. 8.42 The second screw is placed across the sacroiliac joint.

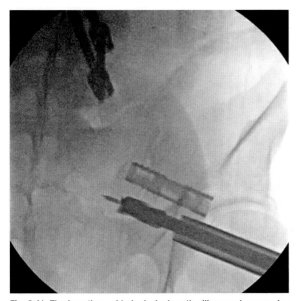

Fig. 8.41 The insertion guide is docked on the ilium, and successive drills create space for insertion of the second screw.

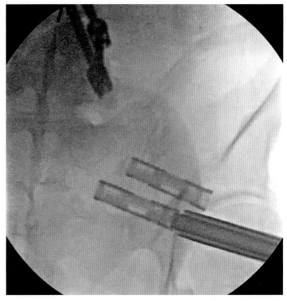

Fig. 8.43 The bone graft is inserted into the second screw.

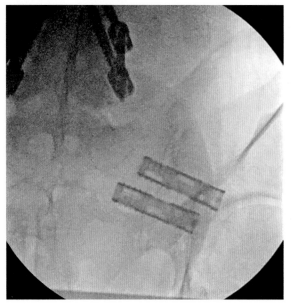

Fig. 8.44 Postoperative imaging of the screw placement in the outlet view.

of other lateral transiliac screw systems. The system uses one Ø13.0-mm main screw with two Ø6-mm integrated side screws, which incorporates three screws into a single trajectory.

TARGETING

The patient is placed in the prone position on the operative table to enable the surgical approach. C-arm fluoroscopy is used to provide imaging during the procedure. Electromyography or similar neuromonitoring may be used to monitor muscles throughout the procedure for increased safety.

Mark the skin at the shadow of the sacrum using a guidewire and marking pen. Mark from the top of the sacrum to the middle of the trochanteric notch. Pull back the tip of the guidewire to the middle of the trochanteric notch along the previous line and draw a perpendicular mark to 1 inch above this location (Figs. 8.46 and 8.47).

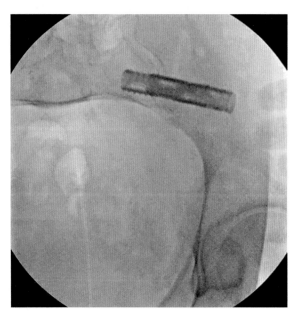

Fig. 8.45 Postoperative screw placement in the inlet view.

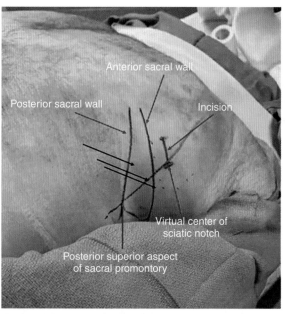

Fig. 8.46 Skin markings using lateral radiography. Note: The pelvis appears to be tilted more anteriorly than is usually seen.

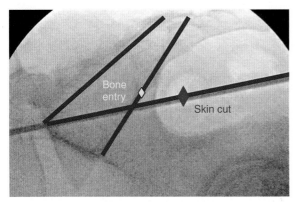

Fig. 8.47 Lateral radiographic view demonstrating how to determine the incision point and desired entry points into the ilium.

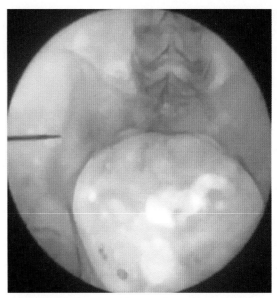

Fig. 8.49 Inlet radiographic view of the guidewire docked.

Make an incision along the 1-inch line. Insert the guidewire lateral to medial through the incision and place guidewire 1.5 to 2 inches superior to the ala of the sacrum. Adjust the C-arm from a lateral to an inlet view to confirm the correct approach (Figs. 8.48 and 8.49).

After the correct entry and approach angle is found, advance the guidewire past the SIJ using a drill. Adjust the C-arm from an inlet view to an outlet view

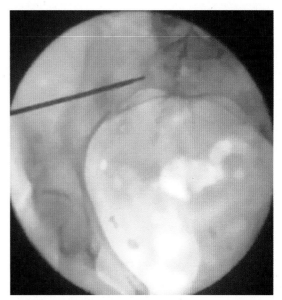

Fig. 8.50 The guidewire is advanced past the sacroiliac joint.

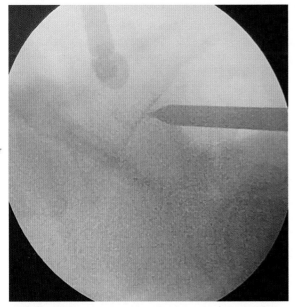

Fig. 8.48 Lateral radiographic view of the guidewire and dilator docked.

and connect the guidewire attachment to the proximal end of the wire if needed. The guidewire has machined slots to help estimate the correct length of the Trident screw to implant. Every slot corresponds to 10 mm (Fig. 8.50).

SCREW PLACEMENT

Select the appropriate length based on the guidewire and assemble a Trident Ø13.0-mm screw onto the introducer sleeve. Insert the Trident screw and introducer sleeve over the guidewire. If using neuromonitoring, place the insulating sleeve over the introducer sleeve at this point. Begin inserting the Trident screw, following the guidewire through tissue to the wall of the ilium (Fig. 8.51).

When the tip of the Trident Ø13.0-mm screw contacts bone, begin screwing into the ilium. Check neuromonitoring (if using) during insertion of the screw. Use the inlet view on the C-arm to align the Trident 13.0-mm screw to allow proper positioning of the Trident Ø6-mm screws (Figs. 8.52 and 8.53).

The correct placement of the screw is determined by feeling when the screw has entered the cortical bone on the posterior wall of the sacrum. The surgeon will feel resistance on passing through the iliac cortical bone of the SIJ and subsequently when the screw passes into the cortical bone of the sacrum. There will be less resistance as the screw passes through the sacral vertebral bodies until the screw approaches the cortical bone of the posterior sacral wall. When this resistance is felt, the screw is turned until the windows of the side openings of the screw are situated so that the side screws will insert into the superior and inferior levels of the sacrum, respectively.

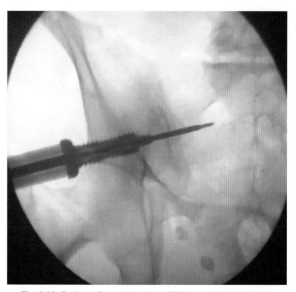
Fig. 8.52 Outlet radiographic view of Trident main screw entry.

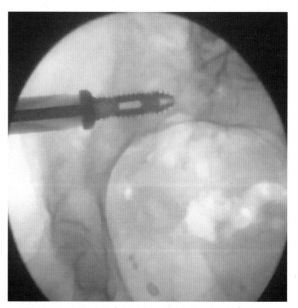
Fig. 8.53 Inlet radiographic view of Trident main screw entry.

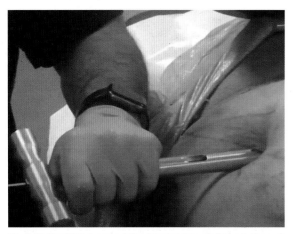
Fig. 8.51 The Trident screw being inserted through tissue to the wall of the ilium.

SIDE SCREW PLACEMENT

Remove the handle, square driver, and guidewire but leave the introducer sleeve in place. Connect the self-retaining side screwdriver to the appropriate length side screw. The self-retaining side screwdriver has a threaded portion at the tip that must be advanced by turning clockwise until the Hexalobe can be engaged. The Hexalobe is self-retaining on the screw when engaged completely. The non–self-retaining side screwdriver is intended to readjust the side screw or to remove it. Insert the side screw and self-retaining driver into the appropriate side opening on the proximal end of the introducer sleeve. The sleeve will guide the side screw into the proper alignment. When the tip of the side screw reaches the ilium, rotate clockwise to insert the side screw into bone. Continue rotating until the side screw stops within the Trident Ø13.0-mm screw. Confirm placement on fluoroscopy. Remove the side screwdriver by pulling it back and then rotating counterclockwise when the Hexalobe is no longer engaged. Repeat side screw steps for the opposing side screw. Confirm placement of the Trident screws on fluoroscopy (Figs. 8.54 to 8.56).

Place the graft delivery sleeve into the introducer sleeve. Use the graft tamp to place bone graft materials into the Trident screw. The main Trident screw includes self-tapping graft collection flutes that reduce the amount of additional biologic agent needed.

Remove the graft tamp and graft delivery sleeve by pulling them out of the introducer sleeve. Remove the introducer sleeve from the Trident Ø13.0-mm screw by turning counterclockwise and pulling it out. Perform typical closure and suture procedures to close the operation site.

REFERENCES

1. Rashbaum RF, Ohnmeiss DD, Lindley EM, Kitchel SH, Patel VV. Sacroiliac joint pain and its treatment. *J Spinal Disord Tech.* 2016;29(2):42-48.
2. Sembrano JN, Polly Jr DW. How often is low back pain not coming from the back? *Spine (Phila Pa 1976).* 2009;34(1):E27-E32.
3. Raj MA, Ampat G, Varacallo M. Sacroiliac joint pain. [Updated 2021 Jul 18]. In: *StatPearls* [Internet]. Treasure Island, FL: StatPearls Publishing; 2021.

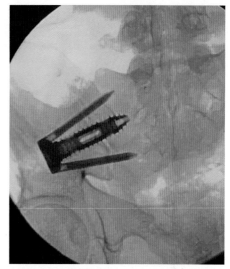

Fig. 8.55 Trident screw placement in the outlet view.

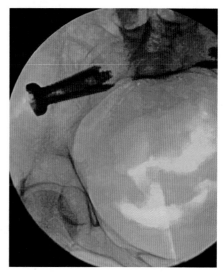

Fig. 8.56 Trident screw placement in the inlet view.

4. Abbasi H, Hipp JA. The assessment of fusion following sacroiliac joint fusion surgery. *Cureus.* 2017;9(10):e1787.
5. Martin CT, Haase L, Lender PA, Polly DW. Minimally invasive sacroiliac joint fusion: the current evidence. *Int J Spine Surg.* 2020;14(suppl):S20-S29.
6. Lorio MP, Polly Jr DW, Ninkovic I, et al. Utilization of minimally invasive surgical approach for sacroiliac joint fusion in surgeon population of ISASS and SMISS membership. *Open Orthop J.* 2014;8(1):1-6.
7. Abbasi H, Storlie N, Rusten M. Perioperative outcomes of minimally invasive sacroiliac joint fusion using hollow screws through a lateral approach: a single surgeon retrospective cohort study. *Cureus.* 2021;13(7):e16517.

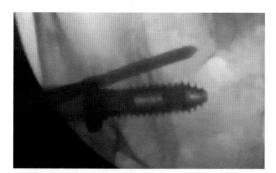

Fig. 8.54 Outlet radiographic view of side screw insertion.

Chapter 9

Measuring Outcomes of Improvement

Meera Kirpekar, Emmanuel Faluade, and Divya Patel

Introduction

Sacroiliac joint (SIJ) dysfunction is a debilitating condition that accounts for approximately 20% of chronic axial lower back pain (LBP). The diagnosis is made by relief of pain after intraarticular block, though it is typically interpreted alongside provocation tests.[1] Despite a prevalence of 10% to 25%,[2] there are currently no efficacious, long-term treatment options for patients with SIJ pain; this may be secondary to inaccurate diagnoses, poor procedural technique, or the subjectivity of pain. Thus, evidence supporting or refuting the efficacy of current treatment modalities is conflicting. The objectives of this chapter are to present the most frequently adopted pain scales for SIJ pain and to discuss the efficacy of common interventions.

Overview of Pain Scales Related to Sacroiliac Joint Efficacy Treatment Studies

OSWESTRY DISABILITY INDEX

Originally published by Jeremy Fairbank in 1980, the Oswestry Disability Index (ODI) is a validated functional measurement for evaluating axial LBP.[1,2] In recent years, it has been extrapolated to measure responsiveness to SIJ pain interventions. The questionnaire produces a score to quantify level of functional disability related to activities of daily living (ADL)s, that is, pain intensity, personal care, lifting, walking, sitting, standing, sleep, sex life, and traveling (Fig. 9.1). Each disability in ADL is scored from 0 to 5, with 0 indicating no pain to 5 indicating the worst pain imaginable. The scores are then added and converted to a percentage of the maximum score of 50. The resulting percentage can be used to measure the level of disability (Table 9.1).

The ODI has historically been a functional assessment tool for axial related back pain but has received growing traction for its utility for SIJ related pain in recent years.[3] A 2015 prospective multicenter clinical study, conducted by Copay and Cher[2] attempted to determine the change in ODI that corresponds to the minimum clinically important difference (MCID), the smallest change in pain that is considered important to patients, for patients undergoing SIJ fusion and compare the values with those already established for lumbar surgeries. A total of 155 participants underwent examination to recruit participants who were experiencing exclusively SIJ-related back pain and who underwent minimally invasive SIJ fusion. These participants were assessed at baseline and 1, 3, 6, and 12 months after joint fusion with postsurgical follow-up assessments using the ODI questionnaire, Health Transition Item (HTI) of the Short Form Health Survey (SF-36), and a postsurgical satisfaction scale. HTI compares current health with health 1 year prior. At 6- and 12-month intervals, patients were asked to rate their level of satisfaction with surgery. These three measures were selected as global assessments of change and as proxy for objective measures of change, essentially pivotal anchors to determine the MCID.

The MCID has been well established for the ODI for patients after lumbar surgery, typically ranging from 7% to 15%. MCID is determined by a series of calculations, including the following: (1) determination of the minimum detectable change (MDC) defined as the smallest change that can be considered above measurement error with 95% confidence, $MDC = 1.96 \times \sqrt{2} \times$ Standard error of measurement (SEM); (2) the average change of the HTI versus the satisfaction scale; (3) the change difference between the average change scores of the HTI versus the satisfaction scale; and (4) the receiver operating characteristic curve

Section 1 – Pain intensity

- ☐ I have no pain at the moment
- ☐ The pain is very mild at the moment
- ☐ The pain is moderate at the moment
- ☐ The pain is fairly severe at the moment
- ☐ The pain is very severe at the moment
- ☐ The pain is the worst imaginable at the moment

Section 2 – Personal care (washing, dressing etc.)

- ☐ I can look after myself normally without causing extra pain
- ☐ I can look after myself normally but it causes extra pain
- ☐ It is painful to look after myself and I am slow and careful
- ☐ I need some help but manage most of my personal care
- ☐ I need help every day in most aspects of self-care
- ☐ I do not get dressed, I wash with difficulty and stay in bed

Section 3 – Lifting

- ☐ I can lift heavy weights without extra pain
- ☐ I can lift heavy weights but it gives extra pain
- ☐ Pain prevents me from lifting heavy weights off the floor, but I can manage if they are conveniently placed e.g. on a table
- ☐ Pain prevents me from lifting heavy weights but I can manage light to medium weights if they are conveniently positioned
- ☐ I can lift very light weights
- ☐ I cannot lift or carry anything at all

Section 4 – Walking

- ☐ Pain does not prevent me walking any distance
- ☐ Pain prevents me from walking more than 2 kilometres
- ☐ Pain prevents me from walking more than 1 kilometre
- ☐ Pain prevents me from walking more than 500 metres
- ☐ I can only walk using a stick or crutches
- ☐ I am in bed most of the time

Section 5 – Sitting

- ☐ I can sit in any chair as long as i like
- ☐ I can only sit in my favourite chair as long as i like
- ☐ Pain prevents me sitting more than one hour
- ☐ Pain prevents me from sitting more than 30 minutes
- ☐ Pain prevents me from sitting more than 10 minutes
- ☐ Pain prevents me from sitting at all

Section 6 – Standing

- ☐ I can stand as long as I want without extra pain
- ☐ I can stand as long as I want but it gives me extra pain
- ☐ Pain prevents me from standing for more than 1 hour
- ☐ Pain prevents me from standing for more than 30 minutes
- ☐ Pain prevents me from standing for more than 10 minutes
- ☐ Pain prevents me from standing at all

Section 7 – Sleeping

- ☐ My sleep is never disturbed by pain
- ☐ My sleep is occasionally disturbed by pain
- ☐ Because of pain I have less than 6 hours sleep
- ☐ Because of pain I have less than 4 hours sleep
- ☐ Because of pain I have less than 2 hours sleep
- ☐ Pain prevents me from sleeping at all

Section 8 – Sex life (if applicable)*

- ☐ My sex life is normal and causes no extra pain
- ☐ My sex life is normal but causes some extra pain
- ☐ My sex life is nearly normal but is very painful
- ☐ My sex life is severely restricted by pain
- ☐ My sex life is nearly absent because of pain
- ☐ Pain prevents any sex life at all

Section 9 – Social life

- ☐ My social life is normal and gives me no extra pain
- ☐ My social life is normal but increases the degree of pain
- ☐ Pain has no significant effect on my social life apart from limiting my more energetic interests e.g. sport
- ☐ Pain has restricted my social life and I do not go out as often
- ☐ Pain has restricted by social life to my home
- ☐ I have no social life because of pain

Section 10 – Travelling

- ☐ I can travel anywhere without pain
- ☐ I can travel anywhere but it gives me extra pain
- ☐ Pain is bad but I manage journeys over two hours
- ☐ Pain restricts me to journeys of less than one hour
- ☐ Pain restricts me to short necessary journeys under 30 minutes
- ☐ Pain prevents me from travelling except to receive treatment

Fig. 9.1 Oswestry Disability Index questionnaire. (From Costa M, Marshman L. Sex life and the Oswestry Disability Index. Spine J. 2015;15(6):1227.)

TABLE 9.1 Oswestry Disability Index Corresponding Score	
Oswestry Disability Index Score (%)	**Description**
0–20	Minimal disability
21–40	Moderate disability
41–60	Severe disability
61–80	Disabled
81–100	Bedbound

From Mehkri Y, Tishad A, Nichols S, et al. Outcomes after minimally invasive sacroiliac joint fusion: a scoping review. *World Neurosurg*. 2022;6:120-132.

approach, in which MCID is the change score that differentiates within each individual group, respectively. In the Copay and Cher[2] study, the ODI change score was statistically associated with the HTI ($r = 0.49$; $P < .0001$) and the satisfaction scale ($r = 0.34$; $P < .0001$). The estimated MCID for ODI resulted in a range between 13% and 15% in this study. This falls within the range of the previously established MCID for lumbar back pain (7%–15%) indicating that ODI may be a valid measure for SIJ disability and that it is sensitive to change in disability.[2]

SHORT FORM HEALTH SURVEY QUESTIONNAIRE

The SF-36 is used as an assessment tool to measure a quality of life after surgery. The SF-36 is comprehensive health survey with a total of 36 questions divided into eight categories, including physical functioning (10 items), bodily pain (2 items), role limitations due to physical health problems (4 items), role limitations due to personal or emotional problems (4 items), emotional well-being (5 items), social functioning (2 items), energy/fatigue (4 items), and general health perceptions (5 items).[4] However, the SF-36 is limited by its lack of assessment of sleep quality, which is pertinent when assessing pain interference with ADLs. The score averages for each category range from 0 to 100, with a higher score defining a more favorable outcome. In addition, the SF-36 may include a HTI, which asks participants retrospective questions. For example, they rate their general health compared with 1 year prior, with five categories of choice, "much better," "somewhat better," "about the same," "somewhat worse," and "much worse."[5] Overall the SF-36 can be used in conjunction with other assessment tools, such as the ODI, to better evaluate the efficacy of proposed treatments and pain related disability.[2,4]

VISUAL ANALOG SCALE

The visual analog scale (VAS) is an additional scale used to determine pain intensity. It consists of a line, approximately 100 mm in length, illustrated in Figure 9.2. The left side signifies no pain, and the right side signifies the worst pain imaginable. There are recommended intervals associated with the intensity of pain, which are no pain (0–4 mm), mild pain (5–44 mm), moderate pain (45–74 mm), and severe pain (75–100 mm).[6] The VAS is most beneficial in self-reported pain that ranges across a spectrum of values that cannot easily be directly measured with a singular value.[6]

THE BRIEF PAIN INVENTORY

The Brief Pain Inventory (BPI) is a multidimensional pain inventory that can reliably provide a measure of the effect of pain on an individual's physical and social

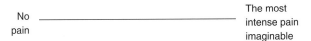

Fig. 9.2 The visual analog scale. (From Benzon H, Raja S, Fishman S, Liu S, Cohen S. *Essentials of Pain Medicine: Pain Assessment*. 3rd ed. Philadelphia: Saunders Elsevier; 2017:29.)

functioning. The BPI consists of a nine-part questionnaire and is available in a short (15 items) (Fig. 9.3) and a long format (32 items). The questions are meant to gauge the severity of pain levels (worst, least, average, and current), the impact of pain on daily functioning in different areas (mood, walking, relationships, sleep, normal work, and general activity), and current treatments with perceived effectiveness of those treatments. The long form of the BPI includes more in-depth questions, including demographic

Brief pain inventory (short form)

Study ID#_____ Hospital#_____
Do not write above this line.

Date: _____

Time: _____

Name: _____
          Last   First   Middle initial

1) Throughout our lives, most of us have had pain from time to time (such as minor headaches, sprains, and toothaches). Have you had pain other than these everyday kinds of pain today?
          1. yes   2. no

2) On the diagram, shade in the areas where you feel pain. Put an X on the area that hurts the most.

Right Left   Left Right

3) Please rate your pain by circling the one number that best describes your pain at its **WORST** in the past 24 hours.
| 0 | 1 | 2 | 3 | 4 | 5 | 6 | 7 | 8 | 9 | 10 |
No pain   Pain as bad as you can imagine

4) Please rate your pain by circling the one number that best describes your pain at its **LEAST** in the past 24 hours.
| 0 | 1 | 2 | 3 | 4 | 5 | 6 | 7 | 8 | 9 | 10 |
No pain   Pain as bad as you can imagine

5) Please rate your pain by circling the one number that best describes your pain on the **AVERAGE.**
| 0 | 1 | 2 | 3 | 4 | 5 | 6 | 7 | 8 | 9 | 10 |
No pain   Pain as bad as you can imagine

6) Please rate your pain by circling the one number that tells how much pain you have **RIGHT NOW.**
| 0 | 1 | 2 | 3 | 4 | 5 | 6 | 7 | 8 | 9 | 10 |
No pain   Pain as bad as you can imagine

7) What treatments or medications are you receiveing for your pain?

_____

8) In the past 24 hours, how much **RELIEF** have pain treatments or medications provided? Please circle the one percentage that most shows how much relief you have received.

0% 10% 20% 30% 40% 50% 60% 70% 80% 90% 100%
No   Complete
relief   relief

9) Circle the one number that describes how, during the past 24 hours PAIN HAS INTERFERED with your:

A. General activity:
| 0 | 1 | 2 | 3 | 4 | 5 | 6 | 7 | 8 | 9 | 10 |
Does not interfere   Completely interferes

B. Mood
| 0 | 1 | 2 | 3 | 4 | 5 | 6 | 7 | 8 | 9 | 10 |
Does not interfere   Completely interferes

C. Walking ability
| 0 | 1 | 2 | 3 | 4 | 5 | 6 | 7 | 8 | 9 | 10 |
Does not interfere   Completely interferes

C. Normal work (includes both work outside the home and housework)
| 0 | 1 | 2 | 3 | 4 | 5 | 6 | 7 | 8 | 9 | 10 |
Does not interfere   Completely interferes

E. Relation with other people
| 0 | 1 | 2 | 3 | 4 | 5 | 6 | 7 | 8 | 9 | 10 |
Does not interfere   Completely interferes

F. Sleep
| 0 | 1 | 2 | 3 | 4 | 5 | 6 | 7 | 8 | 9 | 10 |
Does not interfere   Completely interferes

G. Enjoyment of life
| 0 | 1 | 2 | 3 | 4 | 5 | 6 | 7 | 8 | 9 | 10 |
Does not interfere   Completely interferes

Fig. 9.3 The Brief Pain Inventory (Short Form). (From Waldman SW. Pain management. In: *The Evaluation of the Patient in Pain.* 2nd ed. Philadelphia: Saunders; 2011:198.)

information (age, marital status, education), pain history, aggravating and easing factors, treatment and medication, pain quality, and response to treatment.[7,8]

NUMERIC PAIN RATING SCALE

The Numeric Pain Rating Scale (NPRS) is perhaps the most frequently applied scale used to quantify pain intensity in the clinical setting. It is an 11-point numeric scale, ranging from 0 indicating no pain to 10 indicating worst pain imaginable (Fig. 9.4). Although the NPRS is relatively straightforward and efficient, its utility is limited by its incorporation of only one facet of pain. Because of its simplicity, clinicians may not be able to assess the complexity and idiosyncratic nature of the full pain experience.[9]

Measuring the Efficacy of Interventions

LOCALIZED STEROID INJECTION

Although SIJ injection is an invaluable diagnostic tool, its therapeutic efficacy remains controversial. One retrospective analysis[10] studied 49 patients with pain overlying the posterior superior iliac spine and one or more positive provocative SIJ test results (sacral thrust, Patrick's test, Gaenslen's test) who subsequently underwent unilateral, fluoroscopically guided SIJ corticosteroid injection. To measure efficacy of the intervention, NPRS scores were compared at baseline and at 2 and 8 weeks after intervention. The scoring scale ranged from 0 (no pain) to 10 (severe disabling pain), with a successful outcome defined as a greater than 1.7-point decrease. At both 2 and 8 weeks after the procedure, participants demonstrated significant reductions in NPRS scores (6.6 ± 1.9 at baseline; 2.8 ± 1.4 at 2 weeks; 4.0 ± 1.6 at 8 weeks; P <.0001). Given these supportive findings, the authors cited imprecise technique and inaccurate diagnosis of LBP as barriers to widespread application of localized steroid injection.

In another study,[11] 24 patients with chronic SIJ pain (>6-month duration), refractory to conservative medical therapies, were treated with fluoroscopically guided intraarticular injection of 0.5 mL of 2% lidocaine and 10 mg of triamcinolone followed by periarticular injection of 0.3 mL of 2% lidocaine and 5 mg of triamcinolone. Inclusion criteria were at least one positive SIJ pain provocation test result (pressure application to an SI ligament, Gaenslen's test, Patrick's test), at least 50% pain relief for more than 30 minutes after diagnostic block with the aforementioned injectate, and baseline pain scores greater than 4 on the NPRS score for pain. Treatment efficacy was measured with the NPRS, the ODI, and global perceived effect (GPE) scores; GPE was evaluated on a seven-point Likert scale with higher scores indicating increased patient satisfaction. Evaluations were completed preprocedurally and at 2 and/or 4 weeks postprocedurally. Successful treatment was defined as 50% reduction from baseline NPRS score. Results demonstrated decreases in mean NPRS scores of all patients from baseline (mean ± standard deviation [SD], 6.4 ± 1.2) to 2 weeks (2.2 ± 1.1) and 4 weeks (2.3 ± 1.1) after treatment (P <.05). Similarly, there were decreases in ODI scores from baseline (61% ± 15%) to 2 weeks (21% ± 12%) and 4 weeks (23% ± 11%) after treatment (P <.05). Last, with GPE scores of 6 or greater, 79% of patients reported satisfaction with treatment at 4 weeks. Although this study had a relatively small sample size and was intended to compare the efficacy of an alternative technique, it simultaneously attests to the therapeutic efficacy of corticosteroid injections.

Todorov and Batalov[12] implemented similar measures to compare ultrasound-guided versus landmark-guided SIJ injections. Forty-four patients with spondyloarthritic SIJ pain unresponsive to nonsteroidal antiinflammatory drugs and three or more positive SIJ pain provocative maneuvers (iliac gapping, iliac compression, midline sacral thrust, Gaenslen's test, Patrick's test, sulcus test) were randomized to receive ultrasound- or landmark-guided injection of 7 mg betamethasone (1 mL) and 1% lidocaine (1.5 mL). Self-assessments included the VAS (scored from 0 to 10), Roland-Morris Disability Questionnaire (RMDQ; scored from 0 to 24 quantifying functional disability), and Jenkins Sleep Evaluation Questionnaires (JSEQ; scored from 0 to 20 quantifying sleep disturbance).

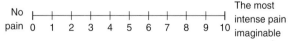

Fig. 9.4 The Numeric Pain Rating Scale. (From Benzon H, Raja S, Fishman S, Liu S, Cohen S. *Essentials of Pain Medicine: Pain Assessment.* 3rd ed. Philadelphia: Saunders Elsevier; 2017:29.)

Assessments were completed before intervention and at 8 weeks after intervention. At the 8-week interval, both groups reported improvements in all outcome parameters. The VAS mean score decreased by 68% and 31% in the ultrasound and landmark groups, respectively, with $P = .004$ representing the significant difference between group responses. RMDQ scores decreased by 46% and 12% in the ultrasound and landmark groups ($P = .031$), respectively. Last, JSEQ scores decreased by 41% and 22% in the ultrasound and landmark groups ($P = .036$), respectively. Again, these results advocate a role for localized corticosteroid injection in the management of SIJ dysfunction.

PLATELET-RICH PLASMA INJECTION

Despite the aforementioned findings, the analgesic response of steroid injection is short term, frequently requiring reinjection and predisposing patients to steroid-related adverse effects. Injections of longer-acting agents, such as the biologic platelet-rich plasma (PRP), have been developed to attempt to overcome these shortcomings.

Singla et al.[13] conducted a randomized control trial to compare ultrasound-guided intraarticular injection of 3 mL of leukocyte-free PRP with 0.5 mL of calcium chloride versus 1.5 mL of methylprednisolone (40 mg/mL) and 1.5 mL of 2% lidocaine with 0.5 mL of saline in 40 patients with moderate SIJ pain (VAS score >3) for at least 3 months. The diagnosis of SIJ pain was confirmed by the presence of three or more positive SIJ provocation tests (sacral thrust, iliac distraction, iliac compression, thigh thrust, Patrick's test, and Gaenslen's test) and imaging consistent with SIJ pathology (radiography, magnetic resonance imaging, or nuclear scan). Outcomes were measured by the VAS, Modified Oswestry Disability Index questionarie (MODQ), and Short Form 12 (SF-12; equally efficient abridgment of SF-36) Health Survey scores. Surveys were performed before the intervention and at 2, 4, 6, and 12 weeks after the intervention. Although the results showed significant reduction in pain intensity (measured by VAS) among all patients from baseline to each follow-up interval, there were no between-group differences in VAS scores at 2 and 4 weeks postinjection. In contrast, 90% of patients in the PRP group reported at least a 50% improvement in VAS at the 12-week interval compared with only 25% of patients

in the steroid group at that time point ($P < .001$). Pain intensity was also lower for the PRP group at 6 and 12 weeks than for the steroid group. Although MODQ and SF-12 scores progressively improved in the PRP group, they decreased in the steroid group at the 12-week follow-up despite an initial uptrend at 2 and 4 weeks. These results suggest PRP injections may have more prolonged analgesic effects and improved functional abilities compared with steroid injections.

Wallace et al.[14] published similar findings regarding the efficacy of PRP injections at 6 months. In this study, 50 patients with more than 1 year of SIJ dysfunction and at least one previous SIJ steroid injection (though not within the last 3 months) underwent ultrasound-guided SIJ injection of 3 mL PRP. The diagnosis of SIJ dysfunction was determined by history and physical examination, imaging, and at least three positive provocative tests (Fortin finger test, Patrick's test, posterior superior iliac spine distraction, Gaenslen's test, pain mapping, thigh thrust test). The primary outcome scale was the ODI, and the secondary outcome scale was the NPRS score. Each measure was completed at baseline and at 1, 3, and 6 months postinjection. Results showed a significant improvement in ODI from baseline to 6 months after injection with the greatest reduction between 2 and 4 weeks. There was also a decrease in NPRS scores. By validating the results of the Singla et al.[13] study with an even longer follow-up interval, this study established the sustainability of PRP injection in SIJ dysfunction.

A retrospective case series by Ko et al.[15] investigated the efficacy of SIJ PRP injections in four patients with SIJ dysfunction; outcome measures included the Short-Form McGill Pain Questionnaire (SFM), NPRS, and ODI. Outcomes were recorded at 1 and 4 years posttreatment. Pooled data at 1-year postinjection showed a 93% reduction in mean SFM ($P < .0001$), an 88% reduction in mean NPRS ($P < .001$), and a 75% reduction in mean ODI ($P < .0001$). The results remained significant at the 4-year follow-up, again substantiating the therapeutic efficacy and longevity of this intervention.

LATERAL BRANCH BLOCKS

Although the previously mentioned studies advocate for SIJ injection, physicians have scrutinized this therapy to address concerns for injectate extravasation through defects in the joint capsule and inadequacy of coverage of the interosseous and dorsal sacroiliac ligaments. As an alternative interventional pain relief strategy, nerve blocks offered much promise. In a double-blind, randomized, placebo-controlled study, Dreyfuss et al.[16] examined the efficacy of sacral lateral branch blocks in 20 healthy, asymptomatic volunteers. During the first session, participants underwent provocation testing through needle probing at the interosseous and dorsal sacroiliac ligaments, dorsal inferior SIJ entry, and capsular distension with contrast. At the second session (1 week later), participants were randomly assigned to receive 0.2 mL of bupivacaine 0.75% or 0.2 mL of normal saline injections at the L5 dorsal ramus and multisite, multidepth S1 to S3 lateral branches. Thirty minutes after the nerve block, provocation tests were repeated. The primary outcome measure in this study was the presence or absence of pain on repeat stimulation. Results showed that only 30% of participants in the active group experienced pain on repeat needle probing and joint entry; however, 80% of participants in the bupivacaine group reported pain with capsular distension. In contrast, 90% to 100% patients in the sham group reported pain with all three repeat provocative tests. These results suggest multisite, multidepth blocks may be 70% effective owing to insufficient coverage of the anterior component of the SIJ. Nonetheless, this study presented nerve blocks as a viable diagnostic and stratification tool in identifying patients with extraarticular SIJ pain who may benefit from lateral branch radiofrequency (RF) neurotomy.

RADIOFREQUENCY ABLATION

Radiofrequency ablation (RFA) is typically considered in patients who have failed the aforementioned therapies. This minimally invasive procedure targets sensory nerves surrounding the SIJ. Dutta et al.[17] compared the efficacy of RF denervation against SIJ injection for the treatment of chronic SIJ pain in a randomized, single-blinded trial. Diagnosis of chronic SIJ dysfunction was defined as 3 months of low back tenderness over the SIJ or three or more positive provocative clinical test results (Gaenslen's test, Patrick's test, Gillet test, thigh thrust test, anterior superior iliac spine compression, and distraction test) and history of a positive response to local anesthetic SIJ injection (at least 80% pain

reduction from baseline for a minimum of 5 hours postprocedure). Using these diagnostic criteria, 30 patients were randomized to receive intraarticular injectate (3 mL solution containing 2 mL of 0.5% bupivacaine and 1 mL of 40 mg/mL methylprednisolone) or pulsed RFA (average temperature, 38°–42°C for a duration 68 ± 12.2 minutes) at the L4 and L5 dorsal rami and S1 to S3 lateral branches. Successful outcomes were defined as a greater than 50% reduction in NPRS score, positive GPE, and at least a five-point reduction in ODI score. The primary outcome measure was NPRS scores, completed at baseline and 15, 30, 90, and 180 days after the procedure. Secondary outcome measures included the GPE and ODI; assessments were completed at baseline and at 90 and 180 days after the procedure. Positive GPE evaluation was indicated by positive response to the following three prompts: (1) "My pain has improved/worsened/stayed the same since my last visit," (2) "The treatment I received improved/did not improve my ability to perform daily activities," or (3) "I am satisfied/not satisfied with the treatment I received and would recommend it to others." Results demonstrated similar NPRS scores at baseline between both groups. At 15 days after the procedure, the mean NPRS scores were more than 50% lower than baseline for both groups ($P = .4265$). Relative to the 15-day follow-up, at 1 month after the procedure, scores remained stable in the steroid injection group from 3.333 to 3.333; in contrast, scores continued to downtrend in the RFA group from 3.200 to 2.933. At 3- and 6-month intervals, pain scores trended upward from the 15-day follow-up for the steroid group to 5.400 and stabilized for the RFA group at 3.200. Mean ODI scores ± SD at baseline were 14.6 ± 4.6 in the steroid group and 15.2 ± 4.3 in the RFA group; by the 6-month interval, the between-group differences were statistically significant with the steroid group scoring 13.1 ± 4.3 and the RFA group scoring 8.0 ± 3.7 ($P = .0017$). Last, GPE responses were positive for 33% of the steroid group and 87% of the RFA group at the 3-month follow-up; at the 6-month follow-up, only 20% of the steroid group, compared to 87% of the RFA group, had positive GPE responses ($P < .05$ at 6 months). With these findings, the authors of this randomized, single-blinded study provided ample evidence for the therapeutic efficacy of RFA in patients with SIJ dysfunction.

Another randomized controlled trial[18] compared the efficacy of L4 to L5 primary dorsal rami and S1 to S3 lateral branch RFA against placebo denervation. Inclusion criteria included axial LBP for more than 6 months, pain over the SIJ refractory to conservative medical therapy, and pain relief of at least 75% for 6 hours after diagnostic SIJ injection. Twenty-eight participants were enrolled and subsequently randomized to cooled RFA or placebo. All patients were reexamined 1 month after the procedure by a physician blinded to interventions. In patients with a positive GPE and greater than 50% pain relief, follow-up examinations were repeated at 3 (intervention was unblinded during this evaluation) and 6 months; virtual appointments were completed every 2 months thereafter to determine duration of effect. In patients who did not have a positive GPE or less than 50% pain relief at the 1-month follow-up, the intervention was unblinded, and patients were offered alternative treatments—conventional, noncooled RFA for failed cooled RFA and crossover to cooled RFA for failed placebo. The primary outcome measure was the NPRS score; secondary outcome measures were the ODI, 20% reduction in opioid use or discontinuation of nonopioid analgesic, and GPE. Successful outcomes included at least 50% reduction in NPRS, positive GPE, and either a 10-point or greater reduction in ODI or a 4-point or greater reduction in ODI coupled with a reduction in analgesic pain medication. Results demonstrated significantly lower NPRS scores in the treatment group than the placebo group (mean $\pm$ SD, 2.4 ± 2.0 vs 6.3 ± 2.4, respectively; $P < .001$) at the 1-month follow-up. Within the RFA group, pain scores were reduced by 60%, 60%, and 57% at 1, 3, and 6 months from baseline, respectively. Eleven participants from the placebo group crossed over with similar reductions in NPRS scores after cooled RFA— 44%, 67%, and 52% at 1, 3, and 6 months, respectively ($P < .001$). With regard to secondary outcomes, the 1-month ODI scores were lower for the treatment arm than placebo (20.9 ± 10.9 vs 43.6 ± 14.0, respectively; $P < .03$). A within-group analysis for the RFA group similarly demonstrated lower ODI scores of 44%, 50%, and 39% at 1, 3, and 6 months, respectively, from baseline ($P < .001$). In contrast, the mean ODI score of the placebo arm was unchanged at 1 month. The crossover placebo group's ODI scores

decreased by 28%, 59%, and 49% at 1, 3, and 6 months. Although the ODI scores did not differ significantly between the initial treatment group and the crossed over placebo group, the initial group did have lower ODI scores at 1 month (20.9 vs 34.3 ± 16.3; $P < .03$). Similarly, for GPE scores, the RFA group had higher scores at 1 month compared with the placebo group (93% vs 21%; $P < .001$). Last, the decrease in analgesic medication intake was greater in the RFA group than in the placebo at 1 month (77% vs 8%; $P < .001$), 3 months (82% vs 0%; $P > .05$), and 6 months (67% vs no data) with similar findings in the crossover placebo group. Regarding duration of analgesia, the treatment group had a mean duration of 5.8 months, and the placebo group reported a mean duration of 0.7 months. In summary, this study further supports the use of RFA in patients with SIJ pain.

Another study[19] examined outcomes of SIJ pain after RFA. Diagnostic criteria for SIJ pain included at least one positive provocative test result (Gaenslen's test, Patrick's test, SIJ shear), reproduction of pain on insertion of needle into the SIJ, and at least 70% improvement in pain after injection of local anesthetics (outcomes measured VAS and pain relief score [PRS]). Patients reporting two or more flare-ups after local blocks, VAS score greater than 50, or pain interfering with ADLs were referred for RFA. VAS scores of 67 patients were recorded before treatment; within 2 hours of treatment; and at 1, 3, and 6 months after treatment to assess longevity of pain relief. Successful outcome was measured as PRS less than 5 or pain reduction of 50% or greater. If patients reported reflares during these intervals, RFA was repeated. Mean VAS scores before intervention were 70.8 ± 12.2 (mean $\pm$SD); 2 hours after RFA, mean scores decreased to 18.8 ± 15.4 ($P < .001$), and PRS was less than 5 for all participants. Thirty patients reported full recovery after initial treatment, with VAS less than 50 and no flares. Effectiveness rates, measured by percentage of PRS less than 5, were 100% immediately after treatment, 73% at 1 month, 46% at 3 months, and 43% at 6 months, with $P < .01$ between 1 and 3 months posttreatment. Thirty-seven patients required multiple treatments; however, of them, 34 reported lower pain scores after each treatment. Based on these results, the authors of this chapter suggested RFA may be considered as viable intervention before surgery.

Additionally, Tinnirello et al.[20] performed a 1-year retrospective observational study comparing Simplicity III (conventional RF) versus SInergy (cooled RF), with both devices being specifically designed for SIJ denervation. Cooled RF has become popularized because of its novel water-cooled technology, exhibiting features of a lower tip temperature in combination with a larger spherical lesions size compared with conventional RF. The study was conducted using 43 patients with SIJ-derived pain refractory to conservative treatment for at least 6 months. The patients were divided between the Simplicity and SInergy groups (21 and 22 patients, respectively). The mean NPRS and ODI scores were determined for each study group to measure outcome for 1, 6, and 12 months postprocedure. The RF procedure was considered a "treatment success" if the patient reported a follow-up NRS score relative to the respective baseline score that was reduced by at least 50% or MCID in ODI scores between baseline and each of the follow-up time intervals with a decrease of 15% or more. Initially, the NRS scores of both groups were equivalent at approximately a score of 7. Throughout the study, the scores of the SInergy group were consistently lower than those of the Simplicity group. However, both groups showed similar patterns of initial dramatic reductions in mean NPRS scores at 1 month. The largest difference in pain reduction occurred at the 6- and 12-month interval scores, which were statistically significant ($P < .01$) between the groups, favoring the SInergy group (NPRS score of 4.3 vs 2.7 at 6 months; 5.1 vs 3.5 at 12 months). Thus, 25% of the Simplicity participants who achieved treatment success at 1 month retained this status at 12 months. In contrast, 68% of SInergy participants who achieved treatment success at 1 month also maintained this success at 12 months. At 12 months, the Simplicity group reported NRS scores that had increased toward baseline values by an average of 50% versus the SInergy group. Twelve-month NRS scores increased relative toward baseline values by an average of 36%. The mean ODI scores of the SInergy group were consistently less than those of the Simplicity throughout the entirety of the 12-month period, with statistically significant ($P < .01$) differences observed at 6 and 12 months. ODI scores illustrated treatment success by showcasing a MCID recognized as 15% or greater with 95% of the SInergy group noting "treatment success" at 1 month and remaining the same at the 6- and 12-month follow-ups. Although 90% of the Simplicity group had ODI score changes that met the MCID criteria at 1 month, there was a noticeable decline of participants who continued to meet the metric each follow-up time visit there afterward (90% at 1 month, 76% at 6 months, 62% at 12 months). This was further appreciated at the 6- and 12-month timeframe, when the SInergy group exceeding those of the Simplicity group by approximately 20% (76% vs 95% at 6 months) and 35% (62% vs 95% at 12 month), respectively. Overall, these data suggest that a greater proportion of patients in the SInergy group experienced superior pain and disability outcomes than those of the Simplicity group at each follow-up, especially at 6 and 12 months. It appears that both conventional RF and cooled RF are effective at treating SIJ pain in the short term, but cooled RF produces significantly longer pain relief that persists. It has been suggested that cooled RF technology allows an interventionalist to create more accurate lesioning of the target nerves because of its larger lesion size, which could explain the longer pain relief.[20]

PERIPHERAL NERVE STIMULATION

Traditionally, patients with SIJ pain unresponsive to conventional progression of treatments (i.e., physiotherapy, antiinflammatory medication, repetitive intraarticular SIJ with local anesthetics and steroids or biologics, neurotomy of the L5–S3 dorsal rami) was were for SIJ arthrodesis or fusion. However, recent research into peripheral nerve stimulation (PNS) presents new opportunities for interventional pain relief. Guentchev et al.[21] extrapolated PNS to the SIJ. Twelve patients with medically refractory SIJ pain were recruited for subcutaneous SIJ neurostimulator implantation. Inclusion criteria included a positive provocative test result (Gillette test, Gaenslen's test, Patrick's test) and a positive SIJ diagnostic test result followed by a steroidal SIJ injection 2 weeks later. Stimulators were implanted after pain recurrence. Outcomes measures included the VAS, ODI, and International Patient Satisfaction Index (IPSI), which were performed before stimulation and at 1 to 2 weeks, 1 to 2 months, 6 months, and 12 months after stimulation. Positive outcome was defined as ISPI score less than or equal to 2. Results demonstrated mean VAS decreased from 9 at baseline to 2.1 at the 2-week interval, 3.8 at the 6-month interval ($P < .0001$), and 1.7 at the 12-month interval ($P < .0001$). ODI decreased from 57% at baseline to 32% at the 2-week interval, 34% at the 6-month interval ($P = .0006$), and 21% at the 12-month interval ($P < .0005$). The IPSI was 1.1 at the 2-week interval, 1.9 at the 6-month interval, and 1.3 at the 12-month interval. The results from this study fostered further investigations into nonsurgical approaches to refractory SIJ pain.

Another study[22] compared percutaneous PNS of medial branch nerves in patients with chronic axial back pain. This was a prospective, multicenter trial that recruited 15 patients with recurrent pain after RFA. Specific inclusion criteria included presence of nonradiating, lumbar LBP for at least 12 weeks, stable analgesic medication use for at least 4 weeks, and baseline pain intensity of at least greater than or equal to 4 on the Brief Pain Inventory Short Form-question 5 (BPI-5). Patients underwent ultrasound- and/or fluoroscopy-guided implantation of percutaneous peripheral nerve stimulators targeting the medial branch nerves overlying the lamina medial and inferior to the facet joint. After 60 days of stimulation, leads were removed, and patients were followed for 5 months. Primary outcomes were daily pain levels and pain medication intake as recorded by patients in weekly diaries; secondary outcomes included the ODI, Brief Pain Inventory-9 (BPI-9), and patient global impression of change. At baseline, average pain intensity was 6.3 (SD, 1.0; BPI-5, scale 0–10). This score decreased to 2.4 ± 1.6 at 2 months ($P < .0001$) and 3.1 ± 1.9 at 5 months ($P < .0001$). Similarly, ODI scores were 43.1 ± 12.7 at baseline, 21.8 ± 13.9 at 2 months ($P = 0.0002$), and 26.1 ± 13.2 at 5 months ($P = .003$). BPI-9 scores were 6.2 ± 1.8 at baseline, 2.4 ± 2.1 at 2 months ($P < .0001$), and 3.2 ± 2.7 at 5 months ($P = .0016$). This report highlights the sustainability and effectiveness of PNS for the treatment of patients with SIJ pain.

ARTHRODESIS

When SIJ pain is refractory to minimally invasive interventions, most physicians recommend SIJ arthrodesis. Buchowski et al.[23] implied arthrodesis improves postoperative function through their case series.

Patients were considered for the arthrodesis only if they had recurrence of SIJ pain after intraarticular SIJ injection and failed all other nonoperative treatments. In total, 20 patients underwent arthrodesis via modified Smith-Petersen or posterior approach.[24] Efficacy of the intervention was measured by performance on the SF-36 and American Academy of Orthopedic Surgeons (AAOS) Modems Instrument. Of the 20 patients, 17 had solid fusion. Fifteen completed the preoperative and postoperative SF-36 (unspecified interval between procedure and completion of postprocedure evaluations), with significant improvement ($P \le .05$) in physical functioning, role physical, bodily pain, vitality, social functioning, role emotional, and neurogenic and pain indices. Although not statistically significant, improvement was also noted in general and mental health ($P < .4706$ and $P < .0604$, respectively). On the AAOS Modems Instrument, patients expressed improvement in the Neurogenic Symptoms Index ($P < .0194$), Pain/Disability Index ($P < .0007$), and Satisfaction with Symptoms Index ($P < .0065$). These results advocate for arthrodesis in patients with SIJ pain unresponsive to conservative measures.

A systematic review reinforcing these findings compared the effectiveness of SIJ fusion.[25] Inclusion criteria were original, peer-reviewed, prospective or retrospective studies with more than two participants. Pertinent exclusion criteria were follow-up less than 1 year and nonsurgical intervention. The review analyzed 16 studies with a total of 430 patients: 131 open procedures and 299 minimally invasive surgical procedures (MIS). Outcome assessment tools were varied among studies; however, many included VAS, SF-36, ODI, NPRS, Majeed scoring system, satisfactory assessment questionnaire, and patient verbal satisfaction. The average durations of follow-up were 60 months for open surgery and 21 months for MIS. Among participants who underwent open surgery, success rates ranged from 20% to 90%; excellent satisfaction ranged from 18% to 100% with a mean of 54% and poor satisfaction, determined by patients indicating they would have rather not had surgery, ranged from 0% to 47%, with a mean of 32%. Among the participants who underwent MIS, excellent satisfaction ranged from 56% to 100%, with a mean of 84%, thus supporting the therapeutic value of this procedure.

Conclusion

Overall, this chapter serves to comment on the most frequently applied pain assessment tools, including the ODI, SF-36, VAS, BPI, and NPRS. Many interventions used to evaluate the efficacy of interventional pain procedures related to SIJ pain incorporate one or more of these scales. As treatment modalities advance from localized corticosteroid or PRP injections to nerve blocks to arthrodesis to even newer methods, it is likely that these assessments will continue to be used to objectively evaluate their efficacies.

REFERENCES

1. Physiopedia. *Sacroiliac Joint Syndrome*. January 8, 2021. Available at: https://www.physio-pedia.com/Sacroiliac_Joint_Syndrome.
2. Copay AG, Cher DJ. Is the Oswestry disability index a valid measure of response to sacroiliac joint treatment? *Qual Life Res.* 2016;25(2):283-292.
3. Mehkri Y, Tishad A, Nichols S, et al. Outcomes after minimally invasive sacroiliac joint fusion: a scoping review. *World Neurosurg.* 2022;6:120-132.
4. Orthotoolkit. *SF-36–OrthoToolKit*. 2021. Available at: https://orthotoolkit.com/sf-36/.
5. Physiopedia. *36-Item Short Form Survey (SF-36)*. May 26, 2020. Available at: https://www.physio-pedia.com/index.php?title=36-Item_Short_Form_Survey_(SF-36)&oldid=239687.
6. Physiopedia. *Visual Analogue Scale*. February 22, 2021. Available at: https://www.physio-pedia.com/index.php?title=Visual_Analogue_Scale&oldid=267491.
7. PainScale. *The Brief Pain Inventory*. (n.d.). Available at: https://www.painscale.com/article/the-brief-pain-inventory.
8. Physiopedia. *Brief Pain Inventory–Short Form*. May 26, 2020. Available at: https://www.physio-pedia.com/index.php?title=Brief_Pain_Inventory_-_Short_Form&oldid=239697.
9. Physiopedia. *Numeric Pain Rating Scale*. May 16, 2020. Available at: https://www.physio-pedia.com/index.php?title=Numeric_Pain_Rating_Scale&oldid=238203.
10. Scholten PM, Patel SI, Christos PJ, Singh JR. Short-term efficacy of sacroiliac joint corticosteroid injection based on arthrographic contrast patterns. *PM R.* 2015;7(4):385-391.
11. Do KH, Ahn SA, Jones R, et al. A new sacroiliac joint injection technique and its short-term effect on chronic sacroiliac region pain. *Pain Med.* 2016;17(10):1809-1813.
12. Todorov P, Batalov A. A comparative study between ultrasound guided and landmarks guided intraarticular sacroiliac injections in spondyloarthritis patients. *Arch Clin Exp Orthop.* 2020;4:001-008.
13. Singla V, Batra RK, Bharti N, Goni NB, Marwaha N. Steroid vs platelet-rich plasma in ultrasound-guided sacroiliac injection for chronic low back pain. *Pain Pract.* 2017;17(6):782-791.
14. Wallace P, Wallace L, Tamura S, Prochnio K, Morgan K, Hemler D. Effectiveness of ultrasound-guided platelet-rich plasma injections in relieving sacroiliac joint dysfunction. *Am J Phys Med Rehabil.* 2020;99(8):689-693.
15. Ko GD, Mindra S, Lawson GE, Whitmore S, Arseneau L. Case series of ultrasound-guided platelet-rich plasma injections for sacroiliac joint dysfunction. *J Back Musculoskelet Rehabil.* 2017;30(2):363-370.
16. Dreyfuss P, Henning T, Malladi N, Goldstein B, Bogduk N. The ability of multi-site, multi-depth sacral lateral branch blocks to anesthetize the sacroiliac joint complex. *Pain Med.* 2009;10(4):679-688.
17. Dutta K, Dey S, Bhattacharyya P, Agarwal S, Dev P. Comparison of efficacy of lateral branch pulsed radiofrequency denervation and intraarticular depot methylprednisolone injection for sacroiliac joint pain. *Pain Physician.* 2018;21(5):489-496.
18. Cohen SP, Hurley RW, Buckenmaier CC, Kurihara C, Morlando B, Dragovich A. Randomized placebo-controlled study evaluating lateral branch radiofrequency denervation for sacroiliac joint pain. *Anesthesiology.* 2008;109:279-288.
19. Ito K. Clinical results of the treatment for sacroiliac joint pain by radiofrequency neurotomy. *Interdisciplin Neurosurg.* 2020;21:1-3.
20. Tinnirello A, Barbieri S, Todeschini M, Marchesini M. Conventional (Simplicity III) and cooled (SInergy) radiofrequency for sacroiliac joint denervation: one-year retrospective study comparing two devices. *Pain Med.* 2017;18(9):1731-1744.
21. Guentchev M, Preuss C, Rink R, Peter L, Wocker E, Tuettenberg J. Treatment of sacroiliac joint pain with peripheral nerve stimulation. *Neuromodulation.* 2015;18(5):392-396.
22. Deer TR, Gilmore CA, Desai MJ, et al. Percutaneous peripheral nerve stimulation of the medial branch nerves for the treatment of chronic axial back pain in patients after radiofrequency ablation. *Pain Med.* 2021;22(3):548-560.
23. Buchowski KM, Kebaish KM, Sinkov V, Cohen DB, Sieber AN, Kostuik JP. Functional and radiographic outcome of sacroiliac arthrodesis for the disorders of the sacroiliac joint. *Spine J.* 2005;5(5):520-528.
24. Smith-Petersen MN, Rogers WA. End-result study of arthrodesis of the sacroiliac joint for arthritis—traumatic and nontraumatic. *J Bone Joint Surg.* 1926;118-136.
25. Zaidi HA, Montoure AJ, Dickman CA. Surgical and clinical efficacy of sacroiliac joint fusion: a systematic review of the literature. *J Neurosurg Spine.* 2015;23(1):59-66.

Index

Page numbers followed by "*f*" indicate figures and "*t*" indicate tables.